VAGINA

# Vagina

## A RE-EDUCATION

Lynn Enright

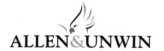
ALLEN&UNWIN

First published in Great Britain in 2019 by Allen & Unwin

Allen & Unwin
c/o Atlantic Books
Ormond House
26–27 Boswell Street
London WC1N 3JZ

Phone: 020 7269 1610
Fax: 020 7430 0916

Email: UK@allenandunwin.com
Web: www.allenandunwin.com/uk

A CIP catalogue record for this book
is available from the British Library.

Internal design by Patty Rennie

Trade paperback ISBN 978 1 91163 001 2
E-Book ISBN 978 1 76063 655 5

Printed and bound by
CPI Group (UK) Ltd, Croydon, CR0 4YY

1 3 5 7 9 10 8 6 4 2

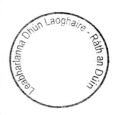

*For my mother, Ann,
and my sisters, Ailbhe and Daire*

# CONTENTS

Introduction                                         1

1   A Sex Re-education                               9

2   The Facts (If We Can Call Them That)            25

3   The Hymen, a Useless Symbol                     45

4   The Clitoris, and How It's Ignored              57

5   The Orgasm, and Why Everything's Normal         73

6   Appearances, and Looking in the Mirror          88

7   Periods, and What Makes Them So Awful          100

8   Pain, As It Applies to Women                   121

9   Fertility, Teaching It and Talking About It    142

10  Getting Pregnant, and What Comes Next          158

11  The Vagina and Menopause                       179

12  Does My Vagina Define Me?                       195

    Acknowledgements                                211

    Resources                                       213

    References                                      217

# Introduction

*I think it's the worst thing we do to each other as women,*
*not share the truth about our bodies and how they work.*
Michelle Obama, *Good Morning America*,
ABC News, 2018

Its very underneathness means the vagina can be overlooked.
Not by the individual, of course: the pulsing of arousal, the
monthly arrival of blood, the sticky discharge, the changing
smells, the unarguable fact that it is the site of new life – all that
means that a woman is never *unaware* of her vagina. But – perhaps due to its position, discreetly tucked away; or perhaps due
to hundreds of years of society controlling women's bodies; or,
most likely, due to a combination of factors – there is a secrecy
surrounding the vagina that afflicts women generally.

As girls we are told, sensibly of course, that it is a private
place; we are urged, really, to ignore it. We call it a 'front bottom', a chirpy if deceitfully vague moniker, and we talk no more
of it until it's time for periods and pregnancy prevention.

There is a fear, it seems, that by presenting a girl with the facts, she will be empowered. And there is sometimes a sense, felt by girls or young women, that they should not be allowed access to that power. I remember as a twelve-year-old hearing that it would be useful to look at my own vagina with a hand mirror. The suggestion came from a representative of Tampax who had come to give a talk at school, and all through the assembly hall echoed murmurs of disgust and ridicule, girls displaying an aversion to the suggestion, signalling to each other that they were horrified at the thought of being so intimate with their own bodies. That night, though, initially compelled because I was the type of studious child who always did her homework, I took a hand mirror – the one that usually sat on the windowsill of my parents' en suite bathroom – and I looked 'down there'. The jolt of arousal was too much; I retreated almost immediately, throwing the mirror aside and pulling up my knickers, depriving myself.

I had been seeking out a biological understanding and, instead of that, or certainly *alongside* that, I had happened upon a deeply erotic experience. Rather than enjoying that undeniable and pleasurable arousal, I was scared: scared of the end of childhood; scared of the new sensation; scared of the possibility of enjoying my sexuality. To masturbate was shameful, something that boys did, not girls, and so I didn't. Not that evening.

Of course, this is just my experience; other girls probably have different memories of the day that they were urged to look at themselves with a hand mirror. Maybe some were able to appraise their vaginas with a dispassionate and scientific eye; maybe others were able to just get on with masturbating, unperturbed by squeamishness, ignorance and the echoing murmurs of disgust. Each girl and woman has a personal and subjective relationship with her vagina – and her sexuality. However, what I think is common is that she exists in a society that discourages her from looking underneath too often; she exists in a society where misinformation about the vagina is rife, where women's sexuality is discouraged and shamed.

It starts early, with the sex education that most of us receive, where there is an emphasis on men's orgasms and male ejaculation. Obviously, when educating teenagers, preventing pregnancy is key, but I remember learning a lot about wet dreams – and wet dreams are about as useless as it gets in terms of procreation. As a young teenager, I was under the impression that boys woke up in sodden sheets each and every morning with dream bubbles featuring topless women floating above their heads. Meanwhile, girls' orgasms or pleasure were never discussed. Basically, in a lot of sex education, the male orgasm is pretty much framed as the point of sex and vaginas are there as a sort of receptacle. And that focus on the male orgasm leads to a situation where girls – and boys – see male sexuality as more important, more dominant than female sexuality.

This misinformation isn't just about attitudes or the way we talk to young people about sex, it's actually right there in the biology too; it's present in the 'facts' we tell people about sex. Close your eyes and conjure up a vagina. Imagine the vagina as represented in one of those anatomical diagrams you once saw in a science or sex ed book. Have you done it? Yes, well that's not what a vagina looks like. Those drawings are inaccurate. They misinform us. They tell us that the labia are symmetrical, when they very rarely are; they depict the vagina – the inner passage – as a sort of open tube (just waiting for a penis perhaps?) when actually the walls touch each other; they illustrate the clitoris as a button without including the crucial clitoral shaft and crura ('legs') that extend beyond the visible nub. They have it wrong.

And that's not where the misinformation ends. Rarely seen in diagrams, but often discussed in relation to young women's vaginas, is the hymen. There is a reason it is not included in diagrams: the hymen – that supposed cling film-like covering that is broken when a girl or woman has sex for the first time – doesn't actually exist in the way we have been told it does. The notion of the hymen isn't erroneous, but it is usually a crescent or ring consisting of folds of membrane that sits slightly inside the vagina. What it looks like and how thick it is differs greatly from woman to woman, vagina to vagina; and for a small minority, it could make intercourse painful or impossible. Crucially, however, it does not – contrary to common belief – act as a kind of seal and it is not 'broken'. Those descriptions of the hymen are nothing more than a misogynistic desire to control young women's sexuality by making their virginity a sort of countable, testable commodity.

So, it's clear that in biology lessons, in sex education classes and in the media, girls are repeatedly handed down inaccurate information. Twenty years on from my own adolescence, girls and young women are still being served up lies about their own bodies, fallacies that serve to obfuscate their understanding of their own vaginas. And this misinformation has consequences.

When information is obscured, harmful myths fill the gaps in knowledge and stigma flourishes. And stigma leads to a situation where a whole lot of girls and women feel bad about their vaginas. Stigma leads to women seeking labiaplasty – the fastest-growing type of cosmetic surgery in the world – to 'correct' asymmetrical labia even though it's perfectly normal to have asymmetrical labia. Stigma leads to women forgoing orgasms because they have never been encouraged to seek them out. Stigma leads to women experiencing health problems because they're too embarrassed to talk to a doctor or healthcare professional. Stigma leads to doctors failing to diagnose and treat endometriosis. Stigma leads to the president of the

United States boasting about grabbing women by the pussy before cutting funding for family planning clinics and abortion providers. Stigma leads to the vagina – and people with a vagina – being undervalued.

We have to smash that stigma. We have to grab that hand mirror and take a long, hard look at what's in our knickers. You can take that literally or metaphorically – it's really up to you. But, either way, what's imperative, what can't be ignored, is the fact that we need to educate, and re-educate, ourselves about our vaginas.

I am cisgender, meaning that my gender identity corresponds with the assumed gender assigned to me at birth. I am a non-disabled neurotypical white woman from Ireland, educated in a Catholic school, currently in a monogamous long-term relationship with a cisgender man. All of that obviously influences how I relate to my own vagina but, throughout the research for this book, I have spoken to a variety of women and people with vaginas, as well as scientists, doctors and experts so that I can represent a broad experience, as well as my own story. I know, however, that I will not be able to tell everyone's story. It is my sincere hope, though, that this book will make it easier for all of us to share our stories. I want to tell my story and I want for you to be able to tell your story.

I know that not everyone who has a vagina is a woman. I know that there are women who do not have a vagina. I recognize that we are living in a time when there is, especially among young people, an increased reluctance to see sexuality and gender as fixed and binary. I think that will only be a good thing for vaginas and people who have them. I know that we are coming up with words and terms to reflect this changing outlook but, as I write this, in late 2018, we are limited. This book generally refers to cisgender girls and women when it says girls and women, largely because I am constrained by the currently available data and research. Similarly, I do not have the data required to consistently include the experiences of trans men and non-binary people in discussions about menstruation, orgasm and pregnancy. I will discuss the trans and intersex experience in Chapter 12 (page 195).

And a quick note on the use of the term 'queer'. Once derogatory, queer has been reclaimed and become standard, especially among young people who don't identify with traditional categories around gender identity and sexual orientation. I use queer when the interviewee or subject identifies as queer. Elsewhere, I use lesbian, gay, bi or LGBTQ+.

In their highly influential 1973 pamphlet 'Witches, Midwives, and Nurses', the feminist authors Barbara Ehrenreich and Deirdre English pointed out that many of the tens of thousands of women who were killed in the witch trials in Europe, the UK and the US in the Middle Ages were midwives.[1]

The medical profession, which was then completely male-dominated (things weren't much better when Ehrenreich and English were writing in the early 1970s), worked alongside the church to target women they saw as competition.

During the three centuries when witch-hunting was commonplace, Ehrenreich and English noted that:

First, witches are accused of every conceivable sexual crime against men. Quite simply, they are 'accused' of female sexuality. Second, they are accused of being organized. Third, they are accused of having magical powers

6

affecting health – of harming, but also of healing. They were often charged specifically with possessing medical and obstetrical skills.

Female healers were accused of providing contraception and abortion; they threatened to imperil and disrupt patriarchal systems of church and medicine – and, for that, they were killed. To know too much about female sexual health has always been seen as an upset to a society that centres the straight male experience.

When Ehrenreich and English wrote the pamphlet, the US was changing – Roe vs Wade, the landmark supreme court ruling that legalized abortion in the US, occurred in the same year as publication. When the pair wrote a new introduction to the treatise in 2010, they reflected on the progress that had been made in the intervening forty years. They spoke about how the urgency to educate women about the menstrual cycle, pregnancy and menopause had perhaps passed, remarking that: 'Today of course, anyone can learn about these things in high school courses, by reading women's magazines, or just by googling.'[2]

Well, yes and no. Ehrenreich and English's new 2010 introduction was written when Barack Obama was president. They didn't know Donald Trump was coming – and with him, threats to abortion rights and the potential undermining of sex education.

And even now, as we approach 2020, googling might result in being served up lies about women's health and sexuality: the Internet might show you Photoshopped images of vulvas; it might suggest that your menstrual cycle is linked to the moon; it might try to sell you a vaginal jade egg. (In fact, it *will* do all of these things.) For clear and unbiased information about women's health, you can't just google.

In the Middle Ages, it was transgressive and mortally dangerous to educate women about their bodies. During the Victorian era, gynaecology became a medical specialization, with male doctors medicalizing women's sexuality, performing unnecessary, sometimes pernicious operations. Throughout most of the twentieth century, the health system remained wretchedly misogynistic, neglecting the safety, sexuality and autonomy of women. And in the late 2010s, we still have more to do: more to learn, more to teach, more to question. We must build on the hard-won gains made by pioneering women like Ehrenreich and English. We must acknowledge the progress that has been made while addressing new challenges posed by the Internet; by tech companies seeking to profit from our bodies; by the rise of the far right.

In this book, I will interrogate the sex education that young people receive. I will address the taboos that continue to silence women and diminish their experiences – taboos around menstruation, female masturbation, miscarriage, menopause and more. I will seek out the information that has not been clear enough: the details of the hymen, the clitoris, the orgasm and the vagina.

Feminism has always, and must always, involve educating women about their own bodies.

CHAPTER ONE

# A Sex Re-education

*Rather than teaching young girls about pleasure, we teach them fear and self-hatred. And rather than teaching young boys about responsibility, we teach them suspicion and slut-shaming.*

Laurie Penny, *Unspeakable Things:*
*Sex, lies and revolution*

I grew up in a home that was relaxed about nudity, a home that was safe and open, with parents who encouraged questioning and learning. But still, we didn't speak of vulvas and vaginas – we spoke of front bottoms. When it came to our own genitalia, we were coy. We were taught to be coy.

My body, throughout childhood and into puberty, was a series of mysteries – some thrilling, some traumatic. I had been told about periods so when blood appeared in my swimsuit one summer at the end of childhood, I knew what it was. But when I saw a white discharge in my pants, I was worried that I was dirty, or sick, or abnormal. No one had ever told me that would happen.

When pubic hair grew, I was prepared, proud even. But when I felt aroused and sensed my clitoris becoming fuller, I was bewildered. I didn't know I had a clitoris – or, more accurately, I didn't know the name for it – until I was well into my teens. My awareness of my body, of my genitalia and my sexual and reproductive organs, was patchy.

I was a child before people had the Internet in their homes. When I was curious or confused, I resorted to looking things up in the big dictionary and the set of dusty encyclopaedias that were kept on a bottom shelf in my parents' bedroom. There was a somewhat informative sex education book in the local library that I never had the courage to officially borrow – but would consult regularly.

By the time my mother sat me down for a sex education talk when I was ten or eleven, I was cognizant of the basics. I knew what menstruation was. I knew how babies were made. I had heard of wet dreams, which fascinated me, even though I had been told they did not apply to me.

I knew little about the intricacies of my own anatomy and almost nothing of the pleasures of which my body was capable. The twenty-minute discussion with my kind but slightly embarrassed mother did not illuminate me in that regard. I implicitly understood that the education pertaining to my own pleasure was more private, an education to be pursued alone.

In the final year of primary school, it was announced that a nurse would be visiting our class for a day. We would have no regular lessons – no long division, no history; there would be no reading aloud, no poems, no learning about mountain ranges. On this allocated day, the nurse would come and tell us about our bodies instead. Attending school on this day was at the discretion of our parents so, if they decided the content of this unusual lesson was unsavoury or unsuitable, we could stay at home and watch daytime TV or catch up on our homework. The nurse's impending arrival was thrilling to me – a break from the monotony of lessons was always welcome and the prospect of talking about sex excited me – but I had a friend who felt differently. She was nervous, embarrassed; she didn't want to sit among her classmates and talk about genitalia and menstruation. She begged her mother to excuse her from the lesson but her mother refused: not, I don't think, because she was especially keen for her daughter to receive a good sex education, but just because of the extra trouble that having a child at home for the day would entail.

On the appointed day, the nurse arrived. My nervous friend coped adequately and all of us girls, even the usually jittery and badly behaved, listened raptly. It felt grown-up, an instruction in adulthood.

It has been more than two decades since that day and I have one particularly clear memory from it. I remember the nurse warning us against the use of tampons – it was healthier, she said, for blood to exit the body; it was wrong, she told us, to capture it inside of ourselves. This image, this propaganda, stayed with me. I even believed it for a while. The rest of the day offered nothing that I hadn't already gleaned from the book in the library, from discussions with my friends or from my mother.

And that was that – we were deemed ready for secondary school. We were ready to turn twelve. We were ready for bras and sanitary towels. That was our sex education: a single day with a woman who planted mistruths among the facts.


It is more than twenty years since I sat in that classroom getting a sex education, and plenty has changed in those years. The

Internet is now freely available – in homes and on children's phones – and, with the Internet, has come an abundance of pornography. It is also clear to me that little girls growing up today are more likely to know the correct anatomical names for their own body parts. When I visited a friend recently, I told her what I was working on: a book about the vagina. Her curly-haired three-year-old daughter overheard me and ran away, into her room, emerging a minute or so later with a book almost as big as she was. She approached me and opened it, pointing to a page that featured an accurate anatomical diagram of the female genitals. This little girl knew the terms for her own anatomy: she knew about vulvas and vaginas. She felt proud of this knowledge – she wanted to share it with me.

My friend explained that she taught her daughter the correct terms – vulva and vagina – so that she is safer, so that she can tell her parents if she is ever touched there, or if she is ever in pain there. This little girl understands that her vulva is a private place, that it is off limits to others – but the fact that it is private does not mean that it has to remain unknown or *private* to herself.

And yet, not as much has changed as I had presumed. I had assumed that sex education must have advanced; I had thought that in the era of the smartphone and sexting and Internet porn, the information we give our children about their bodies and their health and their sexuality would be clearer and more sophisticated. I had thought that the sex education I received in Ireland – a place where the education system was still tethered to the Catholic Church – was an anomaly. I had thought that the UK would have a liberal and sensible approach to sex education that ensured every child and teenager would feel prepared for puberty and knowledgeable about their own body. I was, it turns out, wrong.

In 2017, the children's charity Plan found that one in four girls in the UK felt unprepared for the start of their periods and one in seven did not know what was happening when they began bleeding.[1]

In 2012, the Office for Standards in Education, Children's Services and Skills (Ofsted) carried out a series of inspections relating to the standard of sex education in English schools – the resulting report was titled 'Not yet good enough'.[2] The report stated that:

> Sex and relationships education required improvement in over a third of schools. In primary schools this was because too much emphasis was placed on friendships and relationships, leaving pupils ill-prepared for physical and emotional changes during puberty, which many begin to experience before they reach secondary school. In secondary schools it was because too much emphasis was placed on 'the mechanics' of reproduction and too little on relationships, sexuality, the influence of pornography on students' understanding of healthy sexual relationships, dealing with emotions and staying safe.

When I speak to Lucy Emmerson, director of the UK's Sex Education Forum, a group that works to achieve good relationships and sex education (RSE) for British children and teenagers, she confirms that the standard is patchy: 'I think you would find some examples of schools, where they're teaching RSE in a sex positive way, where they have good lessons on anatomy, where they are talking about pleasure, female as much as male,' she says. But those classrooms are rare. Pushed to guess at the proportion of schools providing an excellent standard of sex education, she hesitates: 'One in ten or one in twenty.'

A new RSE curriculum will be made compulsory in UK schools in September 2020 but, presently, the standard of sex education is random – a lottery. Academies – and schools run by charitable trusts – can, at the time of writing, opt out of teaching sex education completely.

A child who receives a comprehensive and compassionate education about sex and relationships is likely to have done so because of the work and vision of one individual – a teacher, a head teacher, a health worker or someone working in the local council – rather than a joined-up set of countrywide policies. 'It's really going to be a teacher who's made this a specialism, who is confident, who has built up resources for teaching about it, who has looked out for training of their own initiative. It's not going to be a routine thing,' says Lucy Emmerson.

Some children might be lucky; they might have a teacher who believes it's important for them to learn about menstruation, about what a healthy vulva looks like, about masturbation and pleasure. Others might have a teacher who feels awkward or unclear or embarrassed, a teacher who never uses the word 'vagina', who never says 'vulva' or 'clitoris'. 'There are teachers who are unable to utter those words, because they have possibly, in their adult life, never spoken those words out loud,' points out Emmerson. 'Because they got rubbish sex education, they don't use those words in their own personal relationships.'

In Ireland, where I grew up, the Catholic Church is deemed responsible for the dire state of sex education in schools. In Britain, where I live now, there is a sense that some essential *Britishness* might be to blame. 'We're British; we're not good at talking about sex' is a received outlook, and one that contributes to depriving children of information pertaining to their health and sexuality. The fact that RSE is set to become compulsory in British schools is a hugely important shift – and there are some vital changes being made to the curriculum guidelines to better reflect the reality of life for children and teenagers today. The recommendations that children and teenagers are taught about consent – what it is and what it is not – is significant, as is the increased focus on non-heterosexual relationships and sex.

For too long, sex education in the UK (like in most of the rest of the world) has ignored LGBTQ+ sexuality. With so much of the focus on explaining – and preventing – pregnancy, the 'when a man and a woman love each other...' line has been the most consistent. This is set to change with schools being recommended to include 'LGBT-specific content'. This move is especially important given the highly controversial Section 28 clause, introduced as part of the Local Government Act in 1988,[3] which prohibited local authorities and schools from 'promoting' homosexuality. In 1987, Margaret Thatcher told the Conservative party conference: 'Children who need to be taught to respect traditional moral values are being taught that they have an inalienable right to be gay. All of those children are being cheated of a sound start in life. Yes, cheated.'[4] The next year, teachers were banned from talking about same-sex relationships in schools.

Section 28 was repealed in 2000 in Scotland; it took three more years before the Labour government repealed it in the rest of the UK. In the intervening years, some teachers had flouted the rules and taught their students about LGBTQ+ relationships and sex. Many others, however, had given in to the bigotry, with LGBTQ+ children, or those growing up in LGBTQ+ households, feeling alienated and ashamed and confused. Section 28 undoubtedly hampered the progress of gay and trans rights in the UK in the 1980s and 1990s and denied a generation of children access to a compassionate sex education, and so the recommendations that children are given information about LGBTQ+ relationships in all schools after 2020 is an important marker of change and hope.

And yet I don't find myself overly impressed – because, to be frank, the new guidelines are woefully overdue. And they hardly feel radical. They are catching up with a reality that children and young people live every day, rather than presenting a future where teachers and adults truly lead discussions. There is also a worrying vagueness about the training that will be provided to teachers and a lack of clarity on how it will be funded.

And, tellingly, there is a coyness still present. In some respects, the new guidelines are admirable in their ambition – it is vital that we educate our young people about consent, for example – but the advice on how basic facts about bodies and genitals should be taught still feels hazy. In the guidelines I've seen (and it's possible they will change before the 2020 deadline), there isn't clear instruction on whether teachers should use anatomically correct terms – so whether a young child hears words like vulva, vagina and clitoris is probably still going to depend on individual teachers and their individual histories and outlooks.

Even after 2020, parents will be able to withdraw their children from sex education in British schools; and I don't think it's too much of a leap to presume that the parents who opt their kids out of sex education at school are also the parents who will be too embarrassed or disapproving to face the subject head-on at home. That means that after the curriculum has been overhauled, there will still be children attending British schools who will remain ignorant of the correct names for their own genitalia. Children who will be unclear about how sexually transmitted infections are contracted. Children who will be more vulnerable to abuse.

*

Beyond the UK and Ireland, sex education remains patchy and inconsistent, bound up in fears about promiscuity, particularly female or non-heterosexual promiscuity. The South Korean Ministry of Education released sex education guidelines in 2015 that appeared to blame sexual violence on women not going Dutch on dates, suggesting 'women do not pay dating expenses and men want something in return'.[5] Those guidelines have since been revised but gender inequality is still implicit in the country's sex education curriculum, with feminist campaigners working hard to address the problem.

The basics of sex remain a mystery to too many Koreans, even in adulthood, with sex educators in the country pointing out that rudimentary information – like how to put on a condom or how to prevent a pregnancy – is not properly understood by many.[6]

In the United States, meanwhile, only thirteen states actually require that sex education be medically accurate, a bar that seems horrifyingly – almost comically – low. Like in the UK, sex education is a political football in the US and, since Ronald Reagan in the early 1980s, Republicans have generally advocated for sex education that focuses on abstaining from sex until marriage, an approach that leaves teenagers without basic information such as how to use a condom, while enforcing tired and harmful gender stereotypes like female passivity and male sexual aggression.

Under Barack Obama, the Department of Health and Human Services funded comprehensive sex education, which included lessons on contraception, disease prevention, healthy relationships *and* abstinence. Funding for the abstinence-only programmes that proliferated under the George W. Bush administration was cut, and teenage pregnancies declined.[7]

Since Donald Trump was elected president, however, there

have been indications that funding for abstinence-only sex education will be significantly increased.[8] The move to promote and fund abstinence-only sex ed might seem at odds with Trump's own sex life – the boasting about pussy-grabbing; the alleged affair with a porn actress – but his vice president Mike Pence is a long-time advocate for abstinence-based sex ed. As far back as 2002, Pence was claiming that condoms offer 'very, very poor protection against sexually transmitted diseases' – a statement that was fake news before the term fake news had even been invented.[9]

In her 2016 book, *Girls & Sex*, the American journalist Peggy Orenstein addressed the issue of sex education in the US. In a chapter titled 'What If We Told Them The Truth?', she examined the half-truths and flat-out lies teenagers are told in US schools (that latex condoms cause cancer; that the pill is only 20 per cent effective), noting that: 'All together, the US federal government has spent $1.7 billion plus on abstinence-only programs since 1982; that money might as well have been set on fire.'[10]

Orenstein then turned her attention to the Netherlands, a country that has become an international leader in sex education. The Dutch, Orenstein says, 'seem to have it all figured out' – certainly, their teen pregnancy rate is eight times less than that of the US. The UK compares unfavourably to the Dutch too, with roughly five times as many teenage pregnancies.[11] And, beyond the black-and-white of statistics, the Dutch appear to have created a sex education that has love and pleasure and equality at its core: in the Netherlands, sex education is sex-positive.

Sex education is mandatory in Dutch schools, with one-third using resources produced by Rutgers, a non-governmental organization that promotes sexual and reproductive health and rights. (Some councils in England have recently started to use Rutgers materials in schools, too.) In 2018, Ton Coenen, the executive director of Rutgers, outlined the Dutch approach in the *British Medical Journal*:

> In several countries, sexuality education primarily focuses on the negative side: how to avoid an unwanted pregnancy or sexually transmitted infections. In the Netherlands we have evolved a broader approach. How do you engage in a relationship? What is the pleasure in sex?[12]

When I was growing up, the notion of a teacher or an educator explaining that sex was supposed to be pleasurable would have been laughable. It was, I think, sort of assumed that all teenagers desired sex – that was the message I got from TV and films and books, and from the disapproving tone in grown-ups' voices – but nobody was going to help us figure out how to derive pleasure from sex.

The clitoris was never mentioned at school – when I first heard the word, I presumed that it was a slang term as I had never seen it printed in any textbook. For boys, however, it was different; their pleasure was integral to conception and so the male orgasm got a starring role in any discussion of sex. Girls, meanwhile, were tasked with managing its fallout: worrying about pregnancy and how to prevent it.

Lucy Emmerson calls this type of sex education the 'periods, pills and pregnancy' approach. Nobody wins, she says: 'It leaves boys out of the conversation, which is damaging, and it's burdensome to girls.' Good sex education should, she says, challenge gender stereotypes; gender roles and gender inequality should be included in conversations about sex, the body and relationships. And those conversations should begin early. In fact, if we are having honest discussions about the body and anatomy early, it's much more likely that children will feel empowered to ask questions about more complicated notions like gender and consent. That's what good sex education should be: a process that facilitates learning and discussion.

In the Netherlands, sex education at school starts when children are four. This tender age is often seized upon as proof of iniquity by critics, their cheeks reddening: 'Learning about sex at four, how obscene!' But, obviously, four-year-olds are not learning how to put on a condom; they are not learning what sexting is; they are not even learning what sex is. They are learning about aspects of sex and relationships that are appropriate to their age: about the different kinds of relationships – friendships, teacher–pupil, family, romantic. They are learning about their bodies and how to keep them safe.

There are people who will be appalled by a four-year-old knowing the correct words for her anatomy; there are people who will baulk at a young child saying 'vulva' and 'vagina' rather than 'front bottom' or 'girly bits' or 'Minnie' or 'Pookie', or whatever.

There are adults who have a problem with the word 'vagina': a 2015 UK study found that two-thirds of women are embarrassed about saying the word 'vagina'.[13] There are adults who still think that the word 'vagina' is rude, somehow; inappropriate, vulgar, nasty. Advertisements for sanitary towels and tampons don't use the words vagina and vulva, relying on euphemisms like 'V-zone' and 'intimate area' instead. When so many of us are uncomfortable with the word 'vagina', perhaps it's unsurprising that we tend to discourage young children from using the correct terms. But when parents and educators are open and honest about bodies and what they are capable of, they establish a framework that allows for more complicated, more nuanced discussion to take place, too.

When people praise the Netherlands' sex education provision, much is made of the fact that its teen pregnancy rates are so low. The rates are impressive and they make a neat point: being honest about sex with children and teenagers does not lead to increased sexual activity, or increased risky sexual activity, despite what critics of sex education might say. Actually, the opposite might be true: a 2017 survey found that Dutch teenagers were having sex for the first time later (aged 18.6) than they were in 2012 (17.1).[14]

Equally striking is how the Dutch model of sex education – with its focus on love and enjoyment and respect – leads to sex that is more pleasurable and enjoyable for teenage girls. A 2005 study found that four out of five Dutch young people described their first sexual experiences as well-timed, within their control and fun.[15] A couple of years earlier, as my friends and I neared the end of our all-girls secondary school education in a medium-sized Irish town, I'm pretty sure that four out of five of us would have described our first sexual experience as strange, or pressured, or bad. And it wasn't just us. When a study looked at the early sexual experiences of 400 American and Dutch women from similar religious and socioeconomic backgrounds attending similar universities, they found that the Americans were more likely to say they'd had sex for the first time because of 'opportunity' or pressure from friends and partners. Meanwhile the young Dutch women were much more likely to report having had sex for the first time within a loving, respectful relationship.[16] They were more comfortable with their own desire than the Americans, and they were more in touch with their own pleasure.

Without good sex education, my friends and I were left to

fend for ourselves. I consulted my library book in childhood and touched myself in the bath, unclear of what exactly I was touching. When I became a teenager, I gleaned information from teen magazines, publications that seemed to have stepped up to the task of educating girls about sex when all the other grown-ups had given up. And I gave my body over to boys. I didn't have a boyfriend during secondary school and I didn't have sex until I was at university, but at school discos and in the dark lanes between suburban housing estates and, later, at nightclubs where the bouncers were lax about checking IDs, I kissed boys and, sometimes, allowed them to touch me, hoping that it would illuminate me about the mystery of my own body. *This* was my sex education: these fumbles, these hands up skirts and down trousers.

Perhaps that's an inevitable aspect of development, perhaps there can even be something joyous about that – I think some teenagers are especially lucky, coming across partners they love, or at least really fancy, early on, discovering previously unknown pleasure on parents' sofas and in the fields behind school. I believe that's possible. I saw that happen to friends and classmates. That happened to me, sometimes.

But I also believe it's possible to feel pressured into giving boys oral sex. I believe it's possible to become pregnant at fifteen and drop out of school forever. I believe it's possible to pretend to like boys when really you like girls, so afraid are you about what your peers or your teachers or your parents will think. I believe it's possible to be raped and to carry on as though nothing has happened, because you're frightened that by naming the crime you will prolong the trauma, you will make it worse.

I saw all that happen to friends and classmates, too.

When young people begin to have sex, there might be moments of beauty and pleasure and love and brilliance – but, it seems to me that, without providing good sex education, we are leaving too much to luck, to chance. And the consequences can be dire.

It's not perfect in the Netherlands – more girls than boys report experiencing pain during sex and more girls than boys have difficulty reaching orgasm – but the Dutch seem to have proved that when children receive sex-positive sex education that stresses gender equality within relationships, teen pregnancy rates will drop, teenagers will have sex later and girls will have better, more fulfilling sex.[17]

The ramifications of bad sex education are too big to ignore. When 1000 adult British women were tasked with identifying and naming female genitalia in a 2016 study, hundreds of them failed at the most basic level. Forty-four per cent of the women were unable to identify the vagina; 60 per cent of them could not identify the vulva.[18]

The study was carried out by The Eve Appeal, a UK gynaecological cancer charity, and the findings highlight a harmful ignorance. If women are not familiar with what a normal vulva looks like, how will they know to look out for potentially dangerous changes? If they are unclear about where their vagina is and if they feel embarrassed about saying the word 'vagina' aloud, they might not go to a doctor with problems involving pain or a lack of pleasure or a changing smell.

The study proves that sex education in the UK has not been working; it proves that our squeamishness about naming anatomy has real consequences for adults; and it points up the gender inequality at the heart of the issue: of the 1000 women surveyed, 70 per cent could correctly identify the penis, foreskin and testes.

This seems to say something pretty damning about British women's sex lives, too. Because while it's fair to presume that some of the women who cannot identify a vulva still enjoy sex and experience orgasm – being unable to name a body part doesn't mean you can't derive pleasure from it – the ignorance doesn't bode well. After all, the ability to identify your vagina and your clitoris feels like a fairly basic starting point for good sex.

Good sex education should cover consent, sexting and pornography. It should acknowledge and celebrate LGBTQ+ sex and relationships. It should explore issues surrounding fertility and gender roles. Good sex education should feel complicated at times. But it should also feel pretty basic, sometimes. When almost half of women can't identify the vagina, when teachers feel embarrassed even saying the word out loud, it is pretty clear that we urgently need to get the facts about our anatomy straightened out.

Teachers and doctors are reporting that teenage girls feel concerned that their vulvas aren't as neat or as photogenic as the vulvas they see in pornography.[19] Good and kind and thoughtful teachers and doctors are working hard to reassure those teenage girls that vulvas in porn don't represent the average vulva. But if there was a sex education curriculum that showed girls the variance in vulvas before they came across pornography, perhaps the problem could be avoided in the first place. If children learnt more about sex and their bodies in a safe and compassionate environment, they'd be a whole lot less likely to fall for the lies peddled in most mainstream porn.

We need to be able to say 'vulva' and 'vagina'. And we need to be able to see vulvas and vaginas.

CHAPTER TWO

# The Facts
# (If We Can Call Them That)

*Bodies and silence go both easily and uneasily together.*
Emilie Pine, *Notes to Self: Essays*

The fact that, in 2016, 60 per cent of British women were unable to correctly identify the vulva in an anatomical diagram gives us a pretty clear indication of just how neglected the vulva is. What other part of the body would be so overlooked, so unknown? The pancreas, perhaps. Or the appendix, maybe... But they are different. Because the vulva is *right there*. It is an external body part, not an unseen internal organ.

The vulva – which encompasses the clitoris, the mons pubis, the urethral and vaginal openings, and the outer and inner labia – is a site of smell and desire and blood and discharge. It is a place of vitality, of lust, of life – and yet grown women who have had a vulva their whole lives, feel bewildered by it. So bewildered they can't even identify it.

Plenty of us can't even bring ourselves to *say* vulva. After we grow out of words like 'front bottom', we continue to incorrectly name the vulva, calling it the vagina instead. The word vagina is considered embarrassing and shameful; the word vulva is just *absent*. The American feminist and psychologist Harriet Lerner believes this erasure of the word 'vulva' has serious consequences, calling it a 'psychic genital mutilation'. 'What is not named does not exist,' she argues.[1]

The vagina is the passage connecting a woman's outer sex organs to her womb. It's integral to heterosexual sex and to the delivery of babies, so, over the years, the word 'vagina' has been tolerated, if not celebrated. The vulva – with its clitoris – represents something more taboo than even childbirth and menstruation: female pleasure. It represents an independent female sexuality; it names a place of agency, a place that can exist – happily – unperturbed by a penis. And so the word vulva has been sidelined.

I tend to use 'vagina' instead of 'vulva', and I had always assumed that this misnaming was essentially harmless. There was, I suspected, a pedantry to the term 'vulva' – an I'll-think-you-find tone that I didn't want anywhere near my genitals. I like the word 'vagina'; I like saying it, I like hearing it. I think it sounds stronger than 'vulva'. And yet, when I consider Lerner's theory, I find the notion that we're erasing or diminishing a woman's sexuality plausible. Using 'vagina' instead of 'vulva' is essentially calling everything a woman has been given a hole.

We don't say 'vulva'. And we don't really see vulvas, either. On toilet walls and on school locker doors, on binders and on classroom desks, there are penises and scrotums. In permanent marker and in Tipp-Ex, there are primitive drawings of male genitalia. Female genitalia is overwhelmingly overlooked by teenage doodlers, however – and, even in textbooks, it is largely absent. The internal sexual organs – the uterus and the ovaries – are more likely to be depicted in school books. Ask the average woman to draw you a vulva and she'll more than likely struggle. Ask her to draw you a penis, and she'll sketch you a broadly accurate, if rudimentary, representation within minutes.

It wasn't always this way. In the Middle Ages, the vulva was depicted in art and sculpture, and there are thousands of remaining medieval stone carvings of figures with legs open, proudly showing off their vulvas and vaginas, to be found all over Europe. The vulvas and vaginas are not particularly detailed or anatomically accurate in any of these sculptures – they are generally exaggerated and oversized – and historians don't really know their purpose. Looking at them through a twenty-first-century lens, they do not seem erotic; they seem humorous and cheeky, almost cute, like a sexualized troll doll. The skulls and eyes are outsized, along with the genitalia. It is almost impossible for historians to know how they were intended to be understood at the time when they were created, but the best (if far from conclusive) guess is that they were a symbol of fertility. They are known as Sheela-na-gigs and they can be found in France, Norway and the UK, and there is a particular abundance of them in Ireland, adorning churches, castles, defensive structures and wells.

Our wealth of Sheela-na-gigs was not an attraction we seemed to promote when I was growing up in Ireland. We were keen to talk about the Book of Kells, a lavishly decorated gospel displayed at Trinity College, and international visitors were always told to try Guinness – but the stone carvings of female genitalia were not featured in the tourist board literature. In fact, although the modern discovery (and the naming) of Sheela-na-gigs occurred in the mid-nineteenth century, it is only in recent years that they have been studied seriously. As historian Barbara Freitag writes in her 2004 book on the subject: 'Only in the less puritanical atmosphere of the past few decades have academics and artists turned their interest to Sheela-na-gigs.'[2]

27

Thomas O'Connor, the man who made the first modern discovery of a Sheela-na-gig in a church in Tipperary in 1840, was unimpressed, writing that the 'ill executed piece of sculpture', which promoted the 'grossest idea of immorality and licentiousness', should not be anywhere near a church.[3]

It seems perverse, and almost darkly funny, that a country that has for centuries oppressed women and female sexuality – incarcerating unmarried mothers in institutions and outlawing abortion until a historic referendum in 2018 – should have such an abundance of Sheela-na-gigs. For more than 150 years, they were neglected, or hidden, by outraged and ashamed locals, and now, as Ireland embraces a new feminism, there is an increased focus on the nation's Sheela-na-gigs.

The Sheela-na-gigs were created at a time when midwives were accused of witchcraft, when dying during childbirth was not uncommon. It would be naïve to assume that these carvings were a clear-cut celebration of sex, fertility and womanhood and yet their legacy can surely encompass that sentiment. I like to think of the Sheela-na-gigs as ancient feminist forebears of women everywhere, imparting an important message about the need for the visibility of the vulva. We must discard the squeamishness that surrounds the vulva and the vagina. It is what the Sheela-na-gigs would have wanted.

There is a tendency to think of male and female genitalia as opposites; we are taught to think of gender and sex as strictly binary, and we are taught that biology supports this. Men have a penis and women have a vagina – a hole where a penis goes. But that's only some of the story.

It is estimated that between 0.5 and 1.7 per cent of people (that upper figure is the same proportion of the world's population that has red hair) have some intersex traits, meaning they are born with sex characteristics – genitals, reproductive organs, chromosomal patterns – that do not neatly align with typical binary notions of female and male bodies. The World Health Organization estimates that one in every 2000 babies are born visibly intersex[4] – although some say the figure is more like one in 4500. There has been an inclination for doctors to intervene early in such cases, operating on newborns to make them more clearly 'male' or 'female' but there is, increasingly, a mistrust of this sex-assignment surgery.

Even for the majority of people who are born with typical male and female genitalia, there is a shared beginning: for the first six weeks of a foetus's development, its sexual organs are neither male nor female. The genital tubercle will only develop into either a clitoris or a penis at around week seven. In general, women's and men's genitals have more in common than we have been led to believe.

We have been told that men have a penis while women have a vagina. We have been told that men get hard and women get wet (actually men and women both get hard and both get wet: men produce pre-ejaculate and their penises become engorged with blood; women produce arousal fluid and their clitorises become engorged with blood). We have been told – by sex education, by psychoanalysts, by philosophers, by movies, by porn – that the hard penis goes into the wet vagina. And yes, that's true, of course it is: the vast majority of heterosexual people will have lots of penis-in-vagina sex. But to think of sex only in those terms is wrong. It erases non-heterosexual sex; it promotes a strict and unyielding gender binary that isn't even biologically accurate; and it disregards how at least half of women reach orgasm.

To focus too closely on the vagina (especially as some sort of complement to the penis) does women a disservice. Jean-Paul Sartre said that 'the obscenity of the feminine sex is that of everything which "gapes open". It is *an appeal to being* as all holes are.'[5] But the 'feminine sex' is much more than a hole. It is much more than a vagina. It is a whole vulva.

If we are to properly interrogate the way that women's health and sexuality has been belittled and stigmatized, it is necessary to educate ourselves about our own bodies. We must seek to know more about the vulva, the vagina and the internal reproductive organs. It is a sex education that I did not receive; it is a sex education that so many of us did not receive. It is a sex education that will allow us to disentangle ourselves from the patriarchal myths that have acted as binds and ties.

## *The vulva*

The vulva covers a lot. It is the mons pubis (sometimes called the mons Venus or Mound of Venus) – the fatty flesh that covers the pubic bone. It is the clitoral hood and the clitoris underneath that. It is the labia – the outer labia and the inner labia (sometimes called the labia majora and labia minora). It is the vestibule which is the space between the inner labia. It is the urethral opening, which is small and often hard to see. And it is the opening to the vagina, which is also called the vaginal introitus.

Those are the components that make up a vulva. What a vulva looks like, however, differs from person to person. From puberty onwards, hair grows on the mons pubis and on the outer labia. It grows back to the anus and extends out to the top of the thighs. Hair covers the adult vulva, thinning out after menopause, although many women choose to remove some or all of it at various stages in their lives. Some people will have much more hair than others. There will be variation in colour, depending on skin tone, sexual arousal, age and other factors. Some people will have smaller or larger labia, smaller or larger clitorises. There are significant variations in vulvas but, unless a person is experiencing pain, they can assume that their vulva is healthy and normal, even if it looks different to vulvas seen in porn or rudimentary medical diagrams.

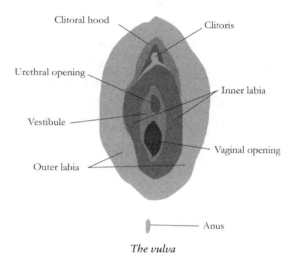

Clitoral hood

Clitoris

Urethral opening

Inner labia

Vestibule

Outer labia

Vaginal opening

Anus

*The vulva*

## The vagina

The muscular tube that leads from the vulva to the uterus is the vagina. It's generally about 7–10 centimetres in length and most of the time the walls of the vagina are squeezed against each other. The vagina can expand to fit a tampon or a finger or a penis, or whatever, but it is not a hole – when I sit in the bath, water does not enter my vagina. The vagina expands during arousal, both lengthways and widthways; it also expands dramatically during childbirth. The vagina is enclosed; it would be impossible to lose anything in the vagina, impossible for anything to make its way further into the body, beyond the vagina, past the cervix. The vagina feels bumpy or ridged to the touch and the vaginal wall is covered with a moist mucous membrane. Some of the moisture present in the vagina is produced in glands (in the cervix or at the opening of the vagina), but moisture seeps through the vaginal walls, too.

The vagina is self-cleaning – the mucous membrane and vaginal flora (bacteria that live in the vagina) keep the vagina healthy by prohibiting the growth of yeast and other organisms. Discharge from the vagina has a slightly acidic taste and smell; this acidity is what prohibits harmful bacteria from developing. The smell and quantity of discharge can vary depending on the stage of the menstrual cycle – and sex or heat or exercise can affect the smell, too. If there is a significant change in the texture or smell of discharge, an infection is likely – and a visit to the doctor is required.

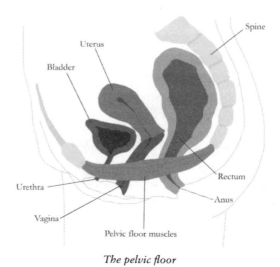

*The pelvic floor*

## *The pelvic floor muscles*

The pelvic floor muscles are the muscles around the vagina, bladder and bowels. Strengthening pelvic floor muscles can help prevent pelvic prolapse (see page 176) and incontinence and can, according to some, improve sex. Pelvic floor exercises, sometimes called Kegels, after the American gynaecologist Arnold Kegel, can be done with or without devices, and are particularly important during and after pregnancy.

## *The Bartholin's glands and the Skene's glands*

The Bartholin's glands are pea-sized bodies located towards the back of the vestibule at either side of the vaginal opening. During arousal, they release fluid into the vagina through ducts. Usually they can't be seen or felt but they can cause pain and become hard if they get blocked or infected, and cysts or abscesses form. Women who have had their Bartholin's glands removed after problems still report 'getting wet' when aroused. It is also possible to be aroused *without* producing fluid in the Bartholin's glands. Fluctuating levels of oestrogen will also influence how much fluid is produced, with people generally producing less at the beginning and end of their menstrual cycles, as well as during breastfeeding and the menopause. The Skene's glands are a set of glands at the opening of the urethra; some women produce fluid here, which is why some women ejaculate or 'squirt' when they orgasm. The type of fluid produced by the Bartholin's glands and Skene's glands – which is sometimes called arousal fluid – is different to cervical fluid.

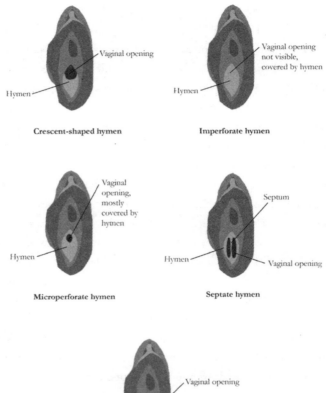

Crescent-shaped hymen

Imperforate hymen

Microperforate hymen

Septate hymen

Ring-shaped hymen

## *The hymen*

The hymen – along with the clitoris and the female orgasm – has been misunderstood and misrepresented for centuries. For this reason, I have chosen to dedicate a whole chapter of this book to it (Chapter 3), examining what it has come to mean in culture and society, and looking at how myths about the hymen can harm girls and women. But here is a basic, biological rundown: the hymen is a mucous membrane along the vaginal opening. It is usually shaped like a ring or a crescent, although some people will have strands stretching across the vagina. In very rare cases, which might require medical intervention, it will appear like a covering. There are significant variations in the hymen from girl to girl and woman to woman, and some people are born without a hymen. Some women's hymens become less noticeable in early adulthood, as hormones change; others will see changes in their hymen after giving birth or reaching menopause. The hymen performs no biological function. It is untrue to say that the hymen is 'broken' the first time a girl or woman has penetrative sex.

## The labia

The outer sides of the outer labia are covered in regular skin. They have pubic hair, although the amount varies from person to person, and they might get spots, eczema, psoriasis or inflamed hair follicles, or any other condition that regularly affects skin. The inner sides are covered in mucous membrane. Generally the outer labia are puffy and fat, and they protect the inner labia and the vestibule. The inner labia have no hair, are thinner than the outer labia and are covered in mucous membrane. They are sensitive with lots of nerve endings. Sometimes, the inner labia sit inside the outer labia but usually they do not; in most people, the inner labia will protrude beyond the outer labia. Often they are unsymmetrical with one side longer than another. The labia change during puberty – getting longer or changing colour, or both – but this is rarely discussed. There is great variation in labia from person to person: a 2018

Swiss study examined 657 white women aged between 15 and 84 years old and found that measurements vary significantly. Some labia measured 2 centimetres in length while others were 10 centimetres.[6]

## The clitoris

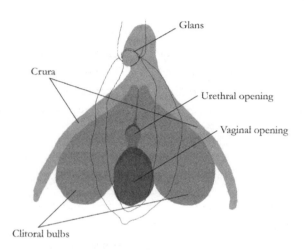

*The clitoris*

I am going to talk about the clitoris in much more detail in Chapters 4 and 5 so, for now, I will stick to a basic description. Beneath the clitoral hood, at the uppermost part of the vulva, is the clitoris. Or, more accurately, is *some* of the clitoris. This visible part, called the glans, varies in size from person to person, ranging from around 0.5 to 3.5 centimetres. The clitoris and the penis have similarities; they have developed from the same embryonic tissue. The glans of the clitoris is, like the glans of the penis, the most sensitive part with thousands of sensory nerve endings. Beyond the glans is the shaft of the clitoris, which then divides into two 'legs', which are known as crura. These crura are inside the body and so are not visible, but they are there, inside the tissue of the vulva, extending back to the vaginal opening. The crura contain corpus cavernosum, or erectile tissue, which fills with blood and becomes engorged during arousal. There are also two clitoral bulbs (sometimes called vestibular bulbs) inside the tissue of the vulva, also made up of erectile tissue, surrounding the vaginal and urinary openings. When a person is aroused, the entire clitoris becomes engorged with blood. Both the crura and the bulbs are covered in muscle and, during orgasm, this muscle can contract, playing a role in the involuntary spasms often felt at that time. The clitoris is the only organ in the human body with the sole purpose of sexual sensation and arousal.

## *The uterus (or the womb)*

The uterus is a small organ with thick and powerful muscular walls, around 7 centimetres long – it's often described as being the size and shape of a small pear. It is hollow, but, like the vagina, its walls press against each other. In pregnancy, this changes and the uterus expands dramatically. In 80 per cent of people, the uterus tips forward, towards the navel, and for 20 per cent of people, it tips backwards.[7] The lining of the uterus, the endometrium, changes significantly during the menstrual cycle: oestrogen and progesterone encourage the endometrium to grow thick in preparation for a fertilized egg, but if there is no pregnancy, oestrogen and progesterone levels will drop and the endometrium will be shed as a period, with the muscular walls contracting.

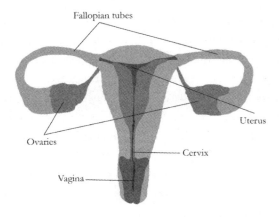

Fallopian tubes

Uterus

Ovaries

Cervix

Vagina

*The reproductive organs*

## *The cervix*

The cervix is the part of the uterus that extends into the vagina, sometimes called the neck of the uterus. It can change position, colour and shape at different stages of the menstrual cycle or when there are hormonal changes in puberty and menopause. When the vagina lengthens during arousal, the cervix is pulled deeper into the body. The opening of the cervix is just a tiny hole, through which menstrual blood or seminal fluid can pass. A finger, penis, menstrual cup or tampon could not fit through it – but, during labour and childbirth, the opening of the cervix dilates to accommodate a baby. There are glands in the cervix that produce cervical fluid, which changes consistency during the menstrual cycle, responding to hormonal changes. At various stages in the cycle, the cervical fluid acts to facilitate or prevent sperm getting past the cervix. Around ovulation, when oestrogen levels are at their highest, the cervical fluid is clear and stretchy like egg white. Cervical screening tests (also called smear tests) check the health of the cells in the cervix –

changes and abnormalities in the cells of the cervix are nearly always caused by the human papillomavirus (HPV) and, if left untreated, these abnormal cells can become cancerous.

## The ovaries and fallopian tubes

The ovaries are almond-sized balls on either side of the uterus. They have two jobs:

1. To store and mature eggs.
2. To produce hormones that control the menstrual cycle.

Eggs develop in sacs in the ovaries called follicles and generally between puberty and menopause a woman will ovulate once every cycle (although there are lots of factors – such as stress, polycystic ovary syndrome (PCOS) and weight fluctuations – that can affect ovulation). When an egg is released from one of the ovaries it travels down the fallopian tube, where it might meet a sperm. If it is fertilized, it will travel to the uterus; if it isn't, it will disintegrate.

## Hormones

Oestrogen and progesterone are the two main female hormones and, until menopause, they are produced in the ovaries. Oestrogen levels fluctuate over the course of the menstrual cycle and some women report feeling happier, more energized and experiencing a higher libido when oestrogen levels are at their highest mid-cycle. Follicle-stimulating hormone (FSH) and luteinizing hormone (LH) are hormones made in the brain: FSH regulates the functions of the ovaries and LH triggers ovulation.

Although testosterone is generally considered to be the male hormone, women produce it too, but most of it is converted into oestrogen.

Those are the facts: I have tried to use language that is plain and clear, language that represents the facts with honesty, without judgement. There will be plenty of polemic; there is an urgent need for polemic. But those are the facts, simple and true.

Those are the facts: some of them I have known since I was a girl, some of them are as obvious to me as the eight times table, as familiar as capital cities.

Those are the facts: some of them I did not know until I started researching this book.

I have lived with a vulva for thirty-five years. I have had sex and menstruated and masturbated and been pregnant and had an abortion. I have had transvaginal ultrasounds and a hysteroscopy and smear tests. Some of the smear tests have shown abnormalities and I have gone back for more smear tests. I have been on the pill; I have used condoms, even when they made my vagina burn. I have had thrush and bacterial vaginosis (BV); I have had a labial cyst. I have monitored my ovulation, testing for LH with sticks I bought in the big pharmacy in the train station on my way home from work. I have experienced infertility. I have had spotting – mysterious bleeding that continues to baffle doctors. I have had tightness, when my vagina seemed stubborn, when it was difficult to insert a tampon or have penetrative sex. I have that tightness, still, sometimes. I have had a vulva for thirty-five years and I still did not know all the facts.

I did not know that the clitoris extended inside the body. I did not know that there was such variation in the length of labia. I did not know what the Skene's glands were.

Even those facts that I have listed so plainly are not the full facts. There are gaps in the facts. There are unknowns in the facts. When I first wrote the paragraphs about the vagina, I included a line about the G spot – describing it as a fleshy area on the front wall of the vagina, which some women find pleasurable to stimulate. I did that because most other books about the vagina include information about the G spot, indicating that many women orgasm when it is stimulated. But then I deleted the line. Because, to me, it didn't feel like a fact. I have a vagina but as far as I can tell, I do not have a G spot, as it has been described in magazines and books. Of course, I am only one person and it would be egotistical, churlish and unethical of me to disregard anatomical fact because it happens not to apply to me. But science doesn't consider the existence of the G spot a fact, either. A 2012 academic review article, published in the *Journal of Sexual Medicine*, with the title 'Is the female G-spot truly a distinct anatomic entity?' delivered no definite answers, with the experts noting that 'the surveys found that a majority of women believe a G-spot actually exists, although not all of the women who believed in it were able to locate it'.[8]

They concluded:

Objective measures have failed to provide strong and consistent evidence for the existence of an anatomical site that could be related to the famed G-spot. However, reliable reports and anecdotal testimonials of the existence of a highly sensitive area in the distal anterior vaginal wall raise the question of whether enough investigative modalities have been implemented in the search of the G-spot.

So... We don't know. Our facts are not robust. Our facts are not fully factual.

*I* think the idea of the G spot was seized upon by a misogynistic media because it encourages women who do not orgasm through penetrative sex to think of themselves as somehow defective, rather than prompting them to question the predominance of heterosexual penis-in-vagina sex that isn't necessarily satisfying for everyone involved.

That is just my opinion. It is not a fact. And I am not a scientist. But I am a woman who has a vagina. I am a woman who doesn't appear to have a G spot. So, based on my experience *and* the science that's currently available, I think the most factually accurate thing to do is to describe the walls of the vagina without including the G spot.

The vulva has been continually let down by science – and by scientists and doctors and anatomists. The full extent of the clitoris was only realized in 1998 and, as we've seen, experts are still arguing over the G spot. However, it is also true to say that there are unassailable facts, clear and straight, that we *do* know about the vagina and the vulva. And yet even when we know the facts – even when there are experts and mothers and grandmothers and public health bodies and feminists that tell us the facts – we are vulnerable to misinformation and manipulation.

With vaginas, it seems, we doubt what we know. With vaginas, we listen to the lies, more than we listen to the truth.

There are doctors carrying out labiaplasty on teenage girls to 'correct' labia that are 'too long' or 'lopsided'. Even though we *know* that the labia are rarely symmetrical and it is normal for them to vary in size.

There are grown women sticking jade eggs up their vaginas

in an attempt to 'boost orgasms, prevent uterine prolapse and regulate periods'.⁹ Even though we *know* that a piece of egg-shaped stone cannot deliver any of goop's promises and is actually more likely to cause harm.

There is a girl standing in the 'feminine hygiene aisle' trying to decide which 'intimate wash' and douche to buy. Even though we *know* that the vagina is self-cleaning and douching can actually increase the risk of infections.

There is a woman feeling despondent, unsatisfied and confused because she can 'only' orgasm through direct clitoral stimulation. Even though we *know* that she is not alone or out of the ordinary: as many as two out of three women require clitoral stimulation to orgasm, or find that clitoral stimulation makes their orgasms more intense.¹⁰

The stigma surrounding the vulva means that knowledge is not disseminated as it should be. Even when some of us know the facts, we are too squeamish, too afraid, too embarrassed to tell everyone. The stigma surrounding the vulva means that knowledge is not as impervious to doubt as it should be. Even when we know the facts, we do not trust what we know.

There are entire industries and systems that flourish and prosper when our knowledge about our vulvas is compromised and undermined: the cosmetic surgery industry; the beauty industry; anyone with a fear of female sexuality; anyone who can profit from that fear.

When Eve Ensler's *The Vagina Monologues* celebrated its twentieth anniversary, I interviewed Ensler about the ongoing impact of the play and theatre project. I enthused about the progress we had made over the last two decades. After all, when she was first publishing the monologues, she encountered resistance: several publishers were reluctant to put out a book with the word 'vagina' in the title. 'We are so much less squeamish now,' I said. 'We have made such significant progress.' She urged caution.

'I think we're less squeamish... absolutely,' she agreed. But then, after the briefest of pauses, she continued, her tone growing urgent:

> Do I think our reproductive rights match our consciousness? No. Do I think patriarchy is still dominant and persistent and stubborn like a horrible virus? Yes, I do. Do I think we move forward and then we move back and then we move forward and then we move back? Yes.[11]

We move forward and then we move back. We get knowledge and then we forget it or we hide it or we lie about it. We *know* where the vulva is. We have known it forever. And yet 60 per cent of women *don't* know where the vulva is.

We are denied facts about our own bodies because female bodies have been ignored and overlooked by science. We are told lies about our own bodies because consumer-goods companies and media organizations can make money from our fearful ignorance. We hide the truth about our own bodies because we are ashamed – of wanting sex, of not wanting sex, of smelling, of bleeding, of orgasming, of not orgasming, of tightness, of looseness, of hair, of pleasure, of pain. We have been taught far more about shame than about our anatomy.

# CHAPTER THREE

# The Hymen,
# a Useless Symbol

*I don't know who*
*invented you – to keep a girl's inwards*
*clean and well-cupboarded.*

Sharon Olds, 'Ode to the Hymen'

For years, I hated the hymen. My hymen, specifically. It caused me embarrassment and shame, acting as an unyielding and stubborn obstacle to sex and real womanhood. As a teenager, when I touched my vulva or attempted to insert tampons, I could find no opening – it was as though the descriptions of anatomy were wrong when applied to me. There was no way in.

I realized that there must be a way *out* because my period arrived when I was twelve. And I could see discharge in my pants. But no prodding and no searching and no longing could help me find that opening, could help me find my vagina.

I knew that the barrier was my hymen. I had been told that the hymen was like a sheath – pierceable and pliable, pulled across the opening of my vagina, ready to be broken when I had sex, or perhaps before, when I used a tampon, or inserted a finger, or even engaged in strenuous activity. But that felt wrong.

The description of the hymen I had been given – from nurses at school, from magazines aimed at teenage girls, from furtive searches on the early Internet – felt wrong.

Now, twenty years later, I *know* that it was wrong. And I know that the misinformation I was given had serious consequences.

'Maybe I broke mine horse riding or when I fell on a fence.' A friend is trying to figure out what became of her hymen. 'Although I never went horse riding as a girl and I don't remember ever falling on a fence.'

She is in her thirties now and about to become a mother, but when she first had penetrative sex as a teenager, she didn't bleed. She doesn't recall the experience as being painful and she says she was only aware of the notion of a hymen because she had encountered it in novels and sex education books.

Several other women I know (women brought up in the 1970s, 1980s and 1990s in the United States, the Middle East, the UK and Ireland) tell me similar stories: they heard about the hymen in school and in books, but as they progressed through their teens – getting their periods; masturbating; giving their bodies over to other teenagers on parents' sofas and at school discos; or experiencing penetrative sex for the first time – it often failed to present itself in the way that they imagined.

'I didn't feel around down there at that age,' says one, recalling her impression of her anatomy during puberty. 'But if I did, I imagined I would have found a tight little piece of skin like a drum surface sheathing my vagina. I assumed it was broken when I lost my virginity.'

That's how a lot of women I speak to *describe* their hymen: a sort of seal, like a piece of translucent sheeting that protects the opening of the vagina, and therefore a woman's purity, waiting to be pierced – usually by a penis.

However, not one of the women I speak to actually confirms ever having encountered her own hymen in the way she would describe it: as in, it wasn't – contrary to expectations, perhaps – a sort of pierceable membrane.

Actually, women's descriptions of their experiences with their hymens seem various – some were unaware of it, some barely aware, and some others experienced difficulty in the same way that I did.

So what's going on here – why are women relaying stories of their hymen so differently? And why are women's descriptions of their own bodies so different to the notion of the taut cling film-like membrane? Is there a disconnect between the imagined hymen and the real, biological hymen? And, if so, why?

Maybe even the word 'hymen' is itself misleading. In Sweden, where the word for hymen is *mödomshinn*, which literally translates as 'virginity membrane', there is a push to rename it *slidkrans*, or 'vaginal corona' in English. Sex education campaigners believe that this renaming of the hymen would remove any unhelpful associations with female purity while simultaneously suggesting a more accurate anatomical understanding – *krans* means 'ring' in Sweden.[1]

Because the thing is: the hymen is not like a drumhead, it is not a tautly pulled skin protecting a girl's vagina. It is – as defined by the anatomy textbook *Gray's Anatomy* – a 'thin fold of mucous membrane situated at the orifice of the vagina'.[2] 'The hymen varies much in shape' from girl to girl, the textbook tells us, but 'when stretched, its commonest form is that of a ring'. Åsa Regnér, a Swedish politician and campaigner seeking to rename the hymen, says, 'Girls have been raised to protect their hymen, not to run, jump, or ride horses. But in reality there is no membrane; rather there are folds of mucous membrane which form a crown around the vaginal opening.'[3]

'It's not a covering,' confirms Adeola Olaitan, a consultant gynaecological oncologist working in private and public practices in London, when I ask her to explain the hymen to me, two decades on from my furtive, fruitless searching. 'In the majority of people it's like a crescent.' Imagine the vagina as a ring, she says, and in most women, the lower part has a crescent – the hymen – partially occluding it. In some cases, the hymen will not be crescent-shaped but will be ring-shaped, too, a circle of tissue sitting just inside the vagina.

In most cases, a vagina – and a hymen – will 'probably accept a finger without any difficulty at all,' Dr Olaitan tells me. 'But there are variations around that.'

So my unyielding, un*open* vagina was a variation? 'What I say to women, is that it's like faces. If you look at faces, it looks a certain way but everyone's face is different, everyone's nose is different, there is no average,' says Dr Olaitan. 'There are variations around a particular theme, and it happens with the genitalia and the hymen.'

It is estimated that around 40 per cent or so of women are born with an 'average' hymen, that crescent shape. Others will have a ring shape. Some may have no hymen or a hymen that is much thicker.[4] Changing hormone levels might mean that the hymen wears away gradually as a girl gets older or it might be stretched through the use of tampons or masturbation. In some cases, remnants of the hymen will be present, even after penetrative sex has occurred and may become more obvious later, after childbirth, for example. The hymen exists in various ways, then – and maybe its very variousness is actually what allows it to take on such intense cultural meanings while remaining mysterious to women.

One woman I speak to – a twenty-six-year-old PR executive called Chloe (not her real name) – tells me she had to have a medical procedure under general anaesthetic when she was nineteen because she wasn't able to have penetrative sex otherwise.

Dr Olaitan points out that a case like this, where a woman is born with what is known as an 'imperforate hymen' is uncommon. 'Needing a surgical intervention to open up the vagina is extremely rare,' she says, but usually a girl or woman will find herself being referred to a specialist if her periods fail to arrive. 'Often it is discovered before people have sex because when people start to have periods, the menstrual blood can't escape so it backs up and fills the womb with blood. It distends the womb, and the womb tries to contract, so young girls will present with severe cramping but no period.'

In Chloe's case, she was able to menstruate, through a very small opening, which meant that her periods were often drawn out, lasting up to two weeks. But sex or even the insertion of a tampon or finger was impossible. 'It was painful and humiliating,' she tells me, 'and it was hard because I had never learnt anything about this. I remember being very confused when I couldn't insert tampons and I thought I was doing something wrong.'

This very unusual imperforate hymen or microperforate hymen (where there is a small hole) is actually quite like the 'stretched membrane/drum head' notion of the hymen that persists in our culture – but even in a situation like Chloe's, that erroneous but persistent description of a sort of cling film-like hymen is wildly unhelpful.

The vagina can feel like a taboo, and the hymen particularly unmentionable, given its connotations of purity. Growing up in a liberal but Catholic home, attending a Catholic school, Chloe had come to associate the hymen with pain, and so it was years – years of experiencing discomfort and confusion; years of not being able to have sex or use tampons – before she sought medical help. It was *supposed* to be difficult, she thought.

The hymen is *not* a film pulled across a girl's vagina *protecting* her virginity, but that is what it has come to be perceived as by many, even by women whose experience of their own hymens, their own vaginas, their own bodies, has told them otherwise. And that notion has been allowed to become so pervasive, in part, I think, because the hymen has no biological function. It serves no purpose and doctors can't be sure as to why it's there. It is only in very rare cases, like Chloe's, that the hymen is of concern to the medical community, and so instead the hymen has become a hugely significant *symbol* in a culture that polices women's sexuality.

Female virginity is seen as a state that must involve a man – and his penis – to be undone. This sense exists in almost every culture, in every religion: being a virgin means to never have had sex – but that sex is usually understood to be penetrative heterosexual sex. The framing of virginity like this disempowers women, allowing their sexuality to be defined by a man's actions – and the hymen then becomes a kind of measurable aspect of that encounter.

In some cultures, there is particular emphasis placed on purity and virginity. In her book on feminism in the wake of the Arab Spring, *Headscarves and Hymens: Why the Middle East needs a sexual revolution*, Egyptian journalist Mona Eltahawy explores the preoccupation with women's purity that exists in Arab cultures. 'Our hymens are not ours,' she says starkly. 'They belong to our families.'[5] A woman who has had sex before marriage will bring shame on her family, she writes, and a woman's virginity is a countable commodity passed on from one family to another, presented to a new husband on a wedding night. Nawal El Saadawi, the Egyptian doctor, writer and feminist activist, puts it like this in her book, *The Hidden Face of Eve: Women in the Arab world*:

> An Arab family does not grieve as much at the loss of a girl's eye as it does if she happens to lose her virginity. In fact if the girl lost her life, it would be considered less of a catastrophe than if she lost her hymen.[6]

El Saadawi was writing in the 1970s but that preoccupation with virginity remains real for many today. Eltahawy points out that it isn't a religious issue, more a cultural one: 'The god of virginity is popular in the Arab world. It doesn't matter if you're a person of faith or an atheist, Muslim or Christian – everybody worships the god of virginity.'

And so some women living in traditional Arab cultures (or in other cultures where virginity is highly valued) – women who have had consensual sex before marriage or have been raped or assaulted – will find themselves in dire circumstances before their wedding night. If a woman is suspected to not be a virgin, her husband will tell his family and she will be punished and shunned. Her family could be ostracized. She might be instantly divorced. There have been particularly heinous cases, in which women who were found to have had sex before marriage were murdered in so-called honour killings.

If a woman does not bleed – which may be the case for a

variety of reasons – her virginity will be questioned, too. El Saadawi says: 'The mere existence of the hymen is not in itself sufficient. [It] must be capable of bleeding profusely, of letting out red blood that can be seen as a visible stain on a white bed sheet the night a young girl is married.'

A Lebanese woman I speak to tells me how young women in more traditional families and communities are encouraged to take some animal or bird blood to their bed on their wedding night: that way they can signal that their virginity has been lost. 'A woman I know did not bleed on her wedding night and that caused a lot of problems for her and her family,' she tells me. Online, you can easily buy a 'fake hymen', which usually consists of a capsule of dye or animal blood that can be inserted into the vagina and will burst during sex.

Some girls and women living in cultures where the hymen is deemed to be vital to a woman's worth have anal sex rather than vaginal sex before marriage – it is not the act of sex that is valued, but the 'intact' hymen. Sometimes, women who have had vaginal sex before marriage resort to a procedure known as hymen reconstruction or hymen repair. At clinics throughout the Middle East and all over the world, there are doctors performing operations designed to make women bleed on their wedding night. Some of the remnants of the hymen, or other tissue present in the vagina, will be fused together, usually with dissolvable sutures a few weeks before the wedding ceremony. And so on the night of her wedding, the woman will bleed when the fused tissue is torn. It is a procedure with no purpose except to perpetuate harmful myths about women's sexuality.

Here in the UK, there are private clinics offering this service and it is occasionally made available on the NHS. Most patients will come from conservative families with Middle Eastern and

Asian backgrounds. Dr Olaitan compares such a procedure, if done for purely cosmetic reasons, to female genital mutilation but stresses that an NHS doctor performing the procedure should have weighed up the benefits for the patient. The thinking goes: although there is no medical indication, if this will save a young woman from being ostracized or mistreated within her family or community, or even killed, then isn't it better to perform it?

For women living in Western cultures, there is less emphasis placed on the hymen, but so-called liberal cultures are still haunted by the hymen and what it represents. It lingers in the way we talk about sex. Virginity is presented as the act of a penis penetrating a vagina, which leaves LGBTQ+ girls and women wondering how to define their first sexual encounters. And when we speak of penis-in-vagina virginity-losing, there is an assumption that the boy or man will orgasm (maybe too soon, the jokes go) whereas the girl or woman will face blood and pain. We don't try to alleviate that pain by discussing the many differences in women's hymens and vaginas; we don't explain enough about lubrication and arousal and how that could make the sex easier and better. We don't point out that the blood could be due to damage in the vaginal wall or tearing because she is not aroused enough.

There is an assumption that a girl or woman will have a bad time the first time she has sex; and actually, in a lot of society, there is even something like a hope that she will.

Recently, when talking about the hymen to a friend, she said: 'What is the hymen's value besides creating discomfort the first time you have sex?' Maybe doctors could routinely examine girls and remove the hymen if it seemed that it would prove problematic for them, she suggested. I thought of Chloe's experience and of my own problems and how much better it would have been if we had felt prepared for that. I thought of how in many cultures, the opposite actually occurs.

'Of course that will never happen,' my friend said after a pause. Because of course we would never trust women with their sexuality like that. Because of course we would not want to be seen as 'encouraging' young women to have sex.

In my own case, my hymen – stubborn and unyielding – became an impediment to sex and relationships as I progressed through my teens. I was embarrassed about how I couldn't seem to find my own vagina and I mainly shied away from relationships and physical intimacy. Occasionally, when I was a bit older, there were situations when kissing progressed to hands up jumpers and down pants and I can still remember holding my breath as another teenager felt for an opening, prodding, trying, before giving up.

I didn't tell a friend. I didn't tell my mother. I didn't tell anyone. *Sex and the City* had arrived on TV in the middle of my teens and I suspected that once I arrived at adulthood, life would be like that: brunch and shopping and writing and friends and sex. But, I lived in a country where abortion would not be legalized for another twenty years. I lived in a town where there were GPs who were known to disapprove of the contraceptive pill and refused to administer it. I could sense that in just a few years, there would be change, but for now, I felt that it was impossible to go to see my GP and say, 'Can you look at my vagina? Can you tell me if there is something wrong?'

Then, when I was nineteen and drunk and asleep in a bed at a party, a man in his twenties who I had met and kissed hours earlier sexually assaulted me. I woke up and my mouth was dry and my pants were filled with blood. I knew it wasn't my period, even as I bled for days afterwards. And I knew something had changed – with my body. Later, weeks later, when I felt brave enough, I put my hand there, and I could feel an opening.

Even now, more than fifteen years later, I don't know what exactly happened that night. The man who touched me without my consent moved away a few weeks later and I have never seen him again. My guess is that he penetrated my vagina – probably with his penis, maybe with his finger, maybe both – and I think that because I was drunk and in a deep sleep, the pain barrier that had always existed before simply wasn't present. He was able to violently open my vagina, pushing away the folds of skin, uninhibited by pain or decency.

Even now, fifteen years later, I don't know what the physiology of my vagina and my hymen had been before that. It remains a mystery. Again, I make guesses: I was, I think, one of those women with thick folds of mucous membrane. I would guess that my hymen occluded my vagina almost completely.

What I do know, what I am certain of, is that an ignorance around the biology of my own body – an ignorance that was encouraged; not maliciously perhaps, but encouraged all the same – meant that I felt I had little autonomy over my own body. And I believe that lack of autonomy, that *ignorance*, left me vulnerable, left me without agency, left me without power.

Why is it that so many of us carry around a notion of the hymen that is different to the biological reality? Is it because we are presented with false information as we grow up? Or is it simply because the hymen differs from girl to girl and so a textbook description will always feel incorrect to some? Perhaps it's a combination of factors: a succession of signs – some nefariously misleading, some benignly confusing – have led us to a place where misinformation surrounds the hymen.

And in that swell of half-truths, cultural and patriarchal

myths have been allowed to flourish. Patriarchal society invests in the notion of the hymen – whether it makes that explicit as in Arab culture; or whether it's a more subtle coercion, like the framing of virginity as something a man takes. And the best way to challenge that is with knowledge. Armed with robust information about our own bodies, women can begin to resist those damaging myths.

# CHAPTER FOUR

# The Clitoris, and How It's Ignored

*When I was a girl we'd never heard of this clitoris. In those days everyone thought it was just a case of in out, in out, shake it all about, stars'd light up the sky an' the earth would tremble. The only thing that trembled for me was the headboard on the bed. But y'see, the clitoris hadn't been discovered then, had it? I mean, obviously, it was always there, like penicillin, an' America. It was there but it's not really there until it's been discovered, is it? Maybe I should have married Christopher Columbus!*

Willy Russell, *Shirley Valentine*

Two teachers, one male and one female, stand in front of a class of ten-year-olds in a school in London. The male teacher is leading a sex education module, and today it is focused on the genitalia. He is using flashcards to teach the lesson, cards that have 'vagina', 'penis', 'testicles', 'outer labia' and other words relating to the female and male genitalia printed on them. He holds up the card that says 'penis'. 'Does this belong with the boy or the girl?' he asks. 'The boy,' the children shout. He affixes the card to a figure of a boy. He repeats the process with the 'vagina' card and the 'testicles' card and the 'outer labia' card, helping the children to amass an understanding of the genitalia. He hesitates when he comes to a card that reads 'clitoris'. He does not hold it up in front of the class. He does not ask the children where it should go. The second teacher looks at him quizzically. He shakes his head as if to say, 'No, we don't do that one.'

There are reasons why a teacher might feel nervous introducing the 'clitoris' card to a classroom of children. Without robust guidelines from the government or adequate support from the school in which he teaches, he might worry that he will find himself in a situation where he is passing on information that is not age-appropriate. Perhaps he is apprehensive about the 'clitoris' card because he is concerned about breaching sex ed protocol; perhaps he is apprehensive because he does not know enough about the clitoris to answer any follow-up questions; perhaps he just feels awkward saying the word 'clitoris'.

There are lots of reasons why that teacher might have skipped straight from 'outer labia' to 'foreskin' that day, but when his female colleague relayed the story to me later, we discussed the omission of the 'clitoris' card in the context of female sexuality being undermined. We were amused by this male teacher who couldn't say 'clitoris', but dismayed, too. Because while it was probably not his intention to stigmatize girls' and women's sexuality, it was surely an outcome. He had, by neglecting the clitoris, contributed to a sense that girls' and women's sexuality is of little importance, a sense that it is an inappropriate topic of discussion in a classroom. The children might not have noticed the omission of the clitoris that day, those ten-year-olds might not have realized there was anything missing, but by misleading them about basic biology, that teacher was doing them a disservice.

This omission of the clitoris is not confined to classrooms. It is not just children who are misled about the clitoris. In the years following the end of World War Two, the entire medical community was given bogus information about the clitoris; namely, that it did not exist.

Since 1858, *Gray's Anatomy* had been the definitive medical textbook, a vital resource, full of detailed anatomical drawings, relied on by doctors around the world. In 1901, the clitoris was included in the textbook for the first time.

In 1947, Dr Charles Mayo Goss, an American doctor who had held positions in the medical departments at Harvard and Yale, became editor of the twenty-fifth edition of *Gray's Anatomy*. He removed the clitoris from the textbook: in the diagram of a woman's sexual and reproductive organs, there was no clitoris. The deletion of the clitoris went unremarked upon and no one is clear on why it occurred. One theory is that Goss was influenced by Sigmund Freud's disparaging attitude towards the clitoris (Freud classed so-called 'clitoral orgasms' as 'immature'[1]). Another guess is that Goss, or someone else working on the edition, simply forgot to include the clitoris. The clitoris was reinstated in later editions of *Gray's Anatomy* but Goss's omission proves that it is not just tongue-tied teachers who have neglected women's sex organs.


Over millennia, the clitoris has been unmentioned, ignored, overlooked, deleted. Significant discoveries have been made, and then seemingly undone, with the clitoris coming into focus at moments throughout history before fading into obscurity again.

The Greco-Roman doctor Claudius Galen made several significant medical discoveries (as well as plenty of inaccurate guesses) during his lifetime in the second century, influencing medicine for the following 1500 years. Regarding the female genitalia, he intuited that, 'All the parts, then, that men have, women have too, the difference between them lying in only one thing, which must be kept in mind throughout the discussion, namely, that in women the parts are within, whereas in men they are outside.'[2]

So there was a sense perhaps, a correct sense even, that the clitoris was homologous to the penis – but this probably had more to do with the prevailing thinking that the female body was an inverted (and inferior) version of the male body more than any genuine understanding of the vulva.

In the Middle Ages, to be a woman who possessed knowledge about the female sexual and reproductive organs was considered a sign of witchcraft – and the female body, including the clitoris (which was not yet called the clitoris), was a target of vicious, deadly misogyny as tens and tens of thousands of women were murdered.

During the Renaissance, the clitoris became a focus of attention, as huge developments in the knowledge of anatomy took place. When the French author and anatomist Charles Estienne undertook a comprehensive series of anatomical investigations and published them in a book, *Dissection of the Parts of the Human Body*, in 1545, he identified the clitoris – but he mistakenly linked its function to urination and stigmatized it by referring to it as the 'shameful member'.[3]

The Italian anatomist Realdo Colombo is often credited with 'discovering' the clitoris, writing in 1559 that 'the love or sweetness of Venus' was 'pre-eminently the seat of women's delight', noting that 'if you touch it, you will find it rendered a little harder'.[4] However, his contemporary Gabriele Falloppio (who identified – and gave his name to – the fallopian tubes) claimed that he had in fact discovered the clitoris some years earlier. (Of course, millions of women had *discovered* the clitoris years and years and years earlier.)

By the seventeenth century, the clitoris was known as the clitoris, and in 1671, Jane Sharp, an English midwife, made a sensible contribution to the discussion, writing that 'the clitoris will stand and fall as the yard doth and makes women lustful and take delight in copulation'.[5] Around that same time, Dutch anatomist Regnier de Graaf was figuring out the fact that the clitoris extends beyond the visible tip and includes the clitoral bulbs and the crura. In 1844, a German anatomist called Georg Ludwig Kobelt conducted an impressively comprehensive study of the clitoris and became the first person to draw detailed anatomies of the inner and outer clitoris.

The discoveries made by de Graaf and Kobelt indicated significant progress, but, though the reality of the clitoris – the full extent of the clitoris, if not the exact dimensions – was realized as early as the seventeenth century, that information did not become common knowledge until much, much later. In 1981, *A New View of a Woman's Body*, an American book by the Federation of Feminist Women's Health Centers, included an illustration of the internal clitoris, in a groundbreaking move to empower women by educating them about their own bodies. But perhaps it is safe to say that the anatomy of the clitoris is still widely unknown. I did not know that the clitoris extended beyond the glans until I began researching this book and I regularly encounter women who have no knowledge of this fact until I tell them.

\*

The urologist Helen O'Connell is one of the key figures responsible for our modern understanding of the extent of the clitoris. Urology is the branch of medicine that focuses on surgical and medical diseases of the male and female urinary tract system and the male reproductive organs – and in 1993 O'Connell became Australia's first female urologist. When she was undergoing her training, she noticed that surgeons took special care to avoid particular nerves and blood vessels to preserve sexual function when removing the prostate in men who had prostate cancer. Preserving sexual function in women undergoing pelvic surgery was more about guesswork – none of the textbooks described the nerve or blood supply to the clitoris.

O'Connell began her own research into the nerve and blood supply of female genitalia, dissecting cadavers and using photography to capture the structure of the clitoris. It became apparent that the entire clitoris – not just the nerve and blood supply – had been underestimated. She told journalists in 1998: 'I thought, Damn! I'm not sure the gross anatomy is correct, either.'6 The clitoris was actually larger than anatomy books had depicted it.

Through O'Connell's work, and the work of other pioneering doctors, activists and researchers, we now have a much clearer idea of the dimensions of the clitoris and how it works. We know that clitorises range from 5 to 12 centimetres in length and swell by 50 to 300 per cent when engorged. We know that the crura extend straight out towards the thighs – but during arousal they curl around the vagina. Following the work of a team of French scientists who carried out the first 3D ultrasound of the stimulated clitoris in 2009, we know how the clitoris interacts with the front wall of the vagina, which means we know more about how the clitoris can be stimulated by penis-in-vagina sex (which could explain why some women report having a G spot).

We are learning all this very belatedly and while there are some practical issues that must be acknowledged – the clitoris is difficult to access as it's covered by bone and tissue and there was historically a lack of female cadavers – much of our ignorance can be put down to the fact that it is women, not men, who have clitorises.

A 2005 academic article co-authored by O'Connell states: 'The anatomy of the clitoris has not been stable with time as would be expected. To a major extent its study has been dominated by social factors.'[7]

As Naomi Wolf notes when discussing the 'Where did it go?' 'What is it for again?' intellectual journey regarding the clitoris in *Vagina: A New Biography*, 'The cultural history of Western anatomy does not reveal any parallel continual misplacement and "forgetting" of the location, role, or function of other organs on the human body.'[8]

It is telling that it took Australia's first *female* urologist to consider the nerve and blood supply of the clitoris. It sounds too simplistic: male doctors didn't care about female bodies, female pleasure and female health. But it is *that* simple.

The penis has been seen as integral. The clitoris has been seen as frivolous, like some sort of decorative, slightly ridiculous accessory – a piece of extravagant costume jewellery worn by feminists.

Similarly, the study of the clitoris has been seen as unserious. It has been presumed that investigating it entails motives that are not strictly scientific. Doctors, psychoanalysts and researchers have been discouraged from pursuing its study. The study of the clitoris has been looked down on, scorned, disparaged; it is a field thought to be unprestigious. As the *Sydney Morning Herald* reported following O'Connell's discovery: 'O'Connell, who spends most of her time treating patients with lower urinary tract problems, was pigeonholed as something of a medical feminist cum sex guru.'[9]

Much of the news and TV coverage at the time of O'Connell's discovery was jokey. It was a subject picked up by panel shows; six straight white male comedians would sit around making jokes in which the lack of knowledge surrounding women's bodies was the punchline.

And while the 1981 publication of *A New View of a Woman's Body* was hailed as significant and O'Connell's work was written about with some degree of seriousness in international broadsheets, many of us missed those announcements entirely and went on presuming that the clitoris was just the visible nub. It's not as though biology textbooks were hauled from schools and amended. It's not as though every GP was instructed to let their patients know that, actually, the clitoris was more extensive than any of us realized.

Since 2016, some French schools have used a 3D model of the clitoris to educate children about their own bodies but the move has not been replicated internationally.[10] Our updated knowledge about the clitoris has not made its way into mainstream thinking in the way that it should have. And, with matters pertaining to the clitoris, that's a pattern we have seen again and again. In 1953, the famed sexologist Alfred Kinsey wrote that, 'Intercourse is not the best means of pleasure for women... the clitoris is the center of female pleasure' – more than six decades on, this is still seen as somehow contentious.[11]

For so long the clitoris has been overlooked – and, worse than that, when it has been awarded attention by the medical and religious communities, it has been considered *controversial*, prompting debate, argument, violence. The information pertaining to it has not been clearly presented without judgement. Instead, it has been made to *mean* something. Often something bad, rarely something good.

This suspicion of the clitoris, this minimizing, has serious consequences. It denies women pleasure: when the clitoris is seen as controversial or bogus or frivolous or unimportant, it means that women's orgasms are viewed similarly. And worse, it allows for a situation in which grave violence is inflicted on the clitoris.

Worldwide, it is estimated that there are 200 million girls and women who have been subjected to female genital mutilation (FGM). Across thirty countries in Africa, the Middle East and Asia, where FGM is concentrated, girls and women have their genitals cut. FGM is classified into four types:

1.  Type 1 is known as a clitoridectomy, where some or all of the visible nub of the clitoris is removed.
2.  Type 2 is known as an excision, where parts of the clitoris and the inner labia are removed (sometimes the outer labia are removed, too).
3.  Type 3 is known as infibulation and involves the vaginal opening being narrowed when a sort of seal – formed by cutting and repositioning the labia – is created. (Deinfibulation refers to the practice of cutting the sealed vaginal opening in a woman who has been infibulated – so that she can menstruate, have sex or deliver a baby.)
4.  Type 4 refers to other harmful procedures to the female genitals, such as pricking, piercing, cutting, scraping or burning the vulva.

Two hundred million women live with the consequences of FGM daily: they are certain to have suffered severe pain and bleeding. Sex is likely to be painful; as is urinating and menstruating. Childbirth can be life-threatening as genital scar tissue does not stretch. It is impossible to say with any accuracy how many girls and women die each year as a result of FGM – deaths are covered up and lied about; and often, if they occur at a later time, they are presumed to be unrelated to the procedure.

When deaths *do* make the news, there is a grim comfort to be had – because at least the issue is being discussed openly. In July 2018, the death of a ten-year-old Somalian girl made international headlines: when Deeqa Dahir Nuur was taken to be cut by a traditional cutter in her village, a vein was severed unintentionally and, two days later, when she was still haemorrhaging, her family took her to a hospital, where she died. The attorney general of Somalia decided to pursue a prosecution, the first of its kind in the country, and Mahdi Mohammed Gulaid, the deputy prime minister, said at the time:

> It is not acceptable that in the 21st century FGM is continuing in Somalia. It should not be part of our culture. It is definitely not part of the Islamic religion.[12]

In a country where 98 per cent of women have undergone FGM (and 65 per cent of women support the practice),[13] that is a powerful statement.

FGM is not endorsed by any one religion; it is not featured in any scripture. It is a cultural practice and is recognized internationally as a violation of the human rights of girls and women. The World Health Organization (WHO) states that 'it reflects deep-rooted inequality between the sexes, and constitutes an extreme form of discrimination against women'.[14]

Feminism – and empowering and educating girls and women

about their reproductive and sexual health – is a crucial line of attack in the global fight against FGM.

There is a growing resistance to FGM even in countries, like Somalia, where it's carried out almost universally. The movement to end FGM must come, and is coming, from all parts of society – including local families and communities and religious and other leaders. The international media as well as international activists, feminists and politicians can play a crucial role, too, as long as they understand that change should begin locally.

Nimko Ali is an FGM survivor who co-founded Daughters of Eve, a UK non-profit organization that campaigns against FGM. 'Solidarity is key,' she tells me, but campaigners in Africa must be allowed to lead the conversation. Ali says:

> Women in Africa have been fighting for years to get the issue of FGM on the agenda and when they did they were not allowed to lead the work. I have only been successful and been able to make change because of the women in Africa who did all the work and set the foundation. These women sadly too often are forgotten.

FGM is illegal in the UK and it is illegal for British citizens to carry out or procure FGM abroad, even in countries where it is legal – but there has never been a successful conviction, even though in 2017 alone, NHS figures showed that 5391 women were treated in relation to FGM in the UK. The majority of these were historic cases but it is estimated that at least 135,000 girls remain at risk in the UK.[15] 'We dismiss FGM as something "other",' says Ali. We do not treat it is as 'an organized crime', which it is.

There is perhaps a reluctance by some to criticize FGM as it is so closely connected with particular cultural and ethnic

communities. There can also be a tendency to ignore it or over-
look it – unless you belong to a culture that practises it. But
some campaigners are keen to point out that British and American attitudes of distaste towards FGM are strikingly modern.
White communities in Europe and America have their own histories of FGM.

Dr A. Renee Bergstrom was three years old and living in a
white Christian community in the Midwest in the US when a
doctor performed a clitoridectomy on her in 1947. She shared
her FGM story publicly in 2016, saying at the time: 'The impe-
tus for my writing is concern regarding increased hatred and
disrespect toward women, other cultures and religions – as if
Christians in the United States had a flawless history.'[16]

Bergstrom was subjected to FGM after her mother noticed
her masturbating and brought her to a local doctor. It is not
known how many girls and women have been subjected to FGM
in the US because it was usually, like in Bergstrom's case, used as
a 'cure' for masturbation, something families and victims were
not keen to talk about. It was a procedure shrouded in secrecy
and shame but it's unlikely that Bergstrom, who is now in her
seventies, is a sole survivor.

In Victorian Britain, the clitoridectomy was a procedure
that enjoyed some popularity, largely due to the endorsement
of Isaac Baker Brown, who was a respected gynaecologist at
the time. In 1858, Baker Brown set up a clinic in Notting Hill
called – and it's a mouthful – the London Surgical Home for
the Reception of Gentlewomen and Females of Respectability
Suffering from Curable Surgical Diseases. There, he performed
clitoridectomies. He also published several books that promoted
FGM – and the procedure, known simply as 'the operation',
was supported by Church of England bishops and newspapers
of the time. Baker Brown saw FGM as a cure for masturbation,

'hysteria', mental illness and 'unfeminine behaviour', a vague category that could include 'distaste for marital intercourse'. Usually paid for by men – husbands and guardians – the operations were expensive, costing the equivalent of more than £10,000 in today's money.[17]

In 1867, his 'operation' was debated by the Obstetrical Society and after it became clear that Baker Brown was occasionally performing FGM on women without the consent of their husbands or male guardians (sometimes it was women themselves who requested a clitoridectomy), he lost his membership. Baker Brown was disgraced and spent some time living in the US, where regulations were less strict. He died in London in 1873.[18]

In America, Baker Brown had a fan in John Harvey Kellogg, who was a medical doctor, nutritionist and inventor. Perhaps best known for inventing corn flakes (along with his brother, Will), he also created a legacy of suppressing and shaming women's sexuality. Kellogg was a member of the Seventh-Day Adventist Church for most of his life and abided by its strict rules. He was married but apparently never consummated his marriage; he was vehemently opposed to masturbation and even sex. He believed that female masturbation was responsible for a range of problems, including mental illness, birth defects and cancer. Kellogg – working as the chief medical officer at a sanatorium run by the Seventh-Day Adventist Church – prescribed certain sleeping positions to discourage masturbation. He advocated for the use of bandages and ties to restrict children from masturbating; when that didn't work, he suggested the use of a cage. In some circumstances, when other methods had failed, he advised a clitoridectomy or the burning of the clitoris with carbolic acid.

The fact that Kellogg is the American doctor who has become particularly associated with clitoridectomies and FGM has, admittedly, probably got something to do with his famous name – he even suggested breakfast cereal could help prevent sexual deviance by keeping sexual organs free of congestion. But his boldness and the strength of his convictions plays a part, too. While other doctors performed clitoridectomies with a degree of discretion, Kellogg, like Baker Brown, was vocal about his support for them.

Operating on the clitoris wasn't just seen as a way to curb masturbation or mental illness. Starting in the late nineteenth century, some European and American doctors began to use FGM to treat so-called sexual dysfunction, too.

If you were *too* sexual as a child – if you masturbated – an operation on the clitoris might be recommended. If you weren't sexual *enough* as an adult – if you didn't orgasm with your husband, say, or weren't much interested in sex – an operation on the clitoris might be recommended. In her book, *Female Circumcision and Clitoridectomy in the United States: A history of a medical treatment*, the academic Dr Sarah B. Rodriguez outlines how, from the late nineteenth century continuing well into the twentieth century, doctors across America began recommending 'female circumcision' (the removal of the clitoral hood) to women who didn't orgasm through penetrative sex with their husbands. It was usually white middle class women who underwent – and even sought out – the surgery, as the more well-off were encouraged to see a good sex life as part of a good marriage. Female sexuality was considered secondary to male sexuality, but writes Rodriguez: 'Once prompted, women were expected to be engaged, interested, and responsive to sex with their husbands.'[19] Sex education in marriage manuals from the 1920s onwards stressed the importance of female orgasm – but this was seen as something bestowed on women by men during intercourse.

In 1927, the European royal, Princess Marie Bonaparte (the great-granddaughter of Napoleon's younger brother, Lucien, and, through marriage, the aunt of Prince Philip, the Duke of Edinburgh), had an operation to move the glans of her clitoris closer to her vaginal opening. She had been complaining about her 'frigidity' for years, finding herself unable to orgasm with any of her male partners during sex. She had discussed the matter with her psychoanalyst (Sigmund Freud himself) but to little avail. The operation to move her clitoris – which reportedly shocked Freud – was not considered a success: unsurprisingly, it did not help Bonaparte reach orgasm.[20] Bonaparte's story is one of wealth and privilege and folly – it is often recounted with a wry and frivolous tone – but it also neatly illustrates the ways in which women's bodies are subjected to violence when men's bodies are seen as dominant and women's bodies are seen as defective. Bonaparte was, like many women of the time, complicit in the FGM inflicted upon her – but that does not make the act any less horrifying.

We know more today about the clitoris and how it functions than we have ever known before. But when a teacher stands in front of children, he is too ashamed, too embarrassed, too uncertain to say the word out loud. He feels that it is too dangerous, too controversial, too daring to say: 'This is the clitoris; it can be pleasurable to touch.'

And I can understand that. I know that uncertainty, that reticence, that squeamishness. I have a clitoris and still I know what it feels like to be unsure of the word; unsure of its power and meaning; unsure about saying it out loud; unsure, even, about touching it or looking at it.

We perpetuate the unsureness with our silences – and with

our acceptance of lies. In 2016, *Australian Men's Health* ran an online article titled: '4 Places That Excite Her More Than The G-Spot.'[21] The piece does not mention the clitoris. Clitoral stimulation is how most women orgasm, most easily and most powerfully. That is a fact overlooked in this particular piece of sex advice as it sets out its stall. 'Her climax is a destination to drive towards together' is a sound opening premise, if a little heavy on the motoring metaphor, but as the reader is encouraged to 'explore four new routes to orgasmland', things get bizarre pretty quickly. Readers are told to find a sexual partner's 'A-spot': 'Follow the front wall of her vagina until just before you reach her cervix. There you'll find her A-spot... Swipe your finger across it like a windshield wiper.'

I flinch when I read that sentence. The thought of anyone fumbling about near my cervix is distinctly off-putting and the windshield-wiper action (why must everything come back to cars?) sounds uncomfortable, even painful. The article was written in response to a study that claimed the G spot didn't exist, but nowhere in the piece is the clitoris mentioned. The cervix is mentioned eight times but the clitoris is not mentioned once. It is erased, overlooked, forgotten about.

When the clitoris is mentioned in men's media, it's often presented as a sort of joke. *It's so hard to find. Am I right?*

But it's not.

It is there, there, there. It is here, here, here. Right there. Right here.

We know where the clitoris is. And we know more about the anatomy of the clitoris now than we ever have. We must not let that knowledge be erased, overlooked, forgotten about.

# CHAPTER FIVE

# The Orgasm, and Why Everything's Normal

*It was Freud who decided there were two kinds of orgasm. What did he know? He wasn't a woman. I would love to get him back here and ask him to explain it.*

Erica Jong, *Playboy* (1975)

Orgasms at their best are wonderful but for a long time, instead of feeling good about them, I felt bad about them.

When I was young, I felt confused about even wanting one. Because the female orgasm serves no reproductive purpose, they were absent from my sex education. I literally didn't know they existed.

And so at first, when aged ten or eleven, I began to experience arousal and desire, I was frustrated by the mystery of my own body. I could sense that this pleasurable sensation, this wanting, was supposed to lead somewhere, but even when I touched myself, I didn't, I couldn't, reach a climax. I remember at school people began talking about masturbation, and one girl said that all boys masturbate but very few girls do. Perhaps she was correct in saying that boys masturbate more than girls: a 2011 American study showed that close to three-quarters of teenage boys report masturbating while just under 50 per cent of girls do – but surely it must be considered that some participants in the study were lying...[1] Certainly, boys are more *encouraged* to masturbate; in lots of cultures, it is seen as a rite of passage. There is a mirthful, if squeamish, acknowledgement that teenage boys frequently masturbate.

Girls' sexuality is more overlooked and so when the subject of masturbation came up among my peers in 1990s Ireland, I remember one girl – a girl a little younger than myself – fixing me with a look and saying, 'Girls who masturbate are sick.'

She wasn't a pious girl and, looking back, I think she was almost daring me to contradict her. I think that if I had told her that I touched myself, maybe she would have admitted that she did, too. Maybe we all did it: some of us had probably been reliably bringing ourselves to orgasm since we were very young, as young as three or four. For others among us, it was perhaps a more recent discovery, this new trick that could allay anxiety, induce pleasure. For the rest of us, masturbation was maybe not regular, not wholly and straightforwardly reliable and pleasurable – but it's likely that the great majority of us had touched ourselves, had attempted to figure out the mystery of our own bodies, even as we faced discouragement and a paucity of information.

And yet, throughout my teens, I remained coy about masturbation. Perhaps that coyness was what meant it stayed a pleasurable but orgasm-free experience. Even after teen magazines and Judy Blume books had reassured me that masturbation was a healthy expression of female sexuality, I was furtive about it, not committing completely to discovering what worked for my body.

The shame began to work on multiple levels – there was a

layering of inadequacy: firstly, I was ashamed of wanting an orgasm. And secondly, I was ashamed of not being able to have an orgasm. Later, as I emerged from my teens, when I began to orgasm from direct clitoral stimulation, I was ashamed of not having the right *kind* of orgasm. I was having sex – heterosexual penis-in-vagina sex with foreplay that included oral sex – at this stage and I felt disappointed that this formula did not result in straightforward orgasm, the way it did for my male partners.

At the time, I did not realize that between 50 and 75 per cent of women cannot orgasm through intercourse alone.[2] I did not know that the simultaneous orgasm was largely a Hollywood myth. When I was nineteen, I still thought that one day, after five to ten minutes of penetrative sex, I might orgasm at the exact same moment as my partner, that we might throw our two heads back in one ecstatic motion, our simultaneous cries reverberating around the room.

Like the hymen, the female orgasm is a biological mystery – its evolutionary purpose remains unclear. Like the hymen, it can differ greatly from person to person. And so, like the hymen, it has been bound up in patriarchal myths. Mistruths and spurious theories seem to take precedence over facts. It feels difficult to even *identify* the facts when we are so unwilling to speak openly and honestly about the vagaries of female orgasms.

To begin to unravel ourselves – and our orgasms – from the misinformation, it's necessary to start at the beginning: what is a female orgasm and what is it not?

Emily Nagoski, the academic and sex educator, provides an excellent overview in her book, *Come As You Are*: '[The] great variety and variability makes orgasm almost impossible to define,' she warns us. 'But when you strip it down to the universal essentials, here's what you get: Orgasm is the sudden, involuntary release of sexual tension.'[3]

Nagoski is careful not to define it as the 'pinnacle of pleasure' because sometimes orgasm does not arise from a pleasurable or enjoyable experience. Women can orgasm during a sexual assault or in their sleep or during exercise; an orgasm is not always a high point. But generally, in consensual sex and masturbation, it is a peak, often a deeply pleasurable and satisfying one. There is a sense of striving for it, of chasing it, and then after it hits, and the sensation spreads through the body, there is a moment of feeling elated then satiated. The average female orgasm lasts seventeen seconds[4] and women can enjoy multiple orgasms in a short space of time in a way that men generally cannot.

The female orgasm is often accompanied by contractions in the pelvis and genitals, they can sometimes be felt as a kind of pulsing, but it would be wrong to simply assume that these contractions *are* the orgasm – it's infinitely more complicated than that: in studies, some women have reported having a strong and satisfying orgasm without displaying the physiological signs.[5]

There are various factors, some difficult to control or quantify, that might affect the quality of the orgasm: how stressed you feel; how physically comfortable you feel; how turned on you feel; where you are in your menstrual cycle; who you are having sex with; whether you are taking antidepressants or have been using alcohol and recreational drugs. It is still unclear as to what makes a person unable to orgasm at all, even though it is estimated that 5 to 10 per cent of women fall into this category.[6]

Also uncertain is the role genetics play in women's ability to orgasm: can our genes explain why some of us can orgasm so much more easily than others? Some scientists think that's highly probable but there isn't a consensus.[7]

There are infinite mysteries that still surround the female orgasm: the fundamental question of what exactly is happening in the brain, and how that correlates to the nerves in the genitals or erogenous zones or the spinal cord, continues to be analysed and debated by scientists. But there are some unassailable truths – perhaps the clearest of which is the fact that, for the majority of women, the most reliable way to reach orgasm is by stimulating the clitoris.

This is not a huge mystery and yet it has been treated as one. Yes, some women can think themselves to orgasm. Some can orgasm by having just their nipples touched. Some wake up from a dream, with a start, orgasming. Some orgasm through penis-in-vagina intercourse. But most women orgasm most reliably through the stimulation of the clitoris. There has been a tendency to unnecessarily complicate this reality, to divide orgasms into vaginal orgasms and clitoral orgasms and blended orgasms, which are said to include both – and to rank those orgasms with the most reliable clitoral orgasms being deemed the least satisfying, the least interesting, the least *mature*.

In heterosexual culture, we have been encouraged to view an orgasm that arises from penis-in-vagina sex as a kind of superior orgasm or proper orgasm. We are constantly presented with the notion – in films, in porn, in women's magazines – that women are able to (or will be able to once they put in the effort) orgasm through penetrative intercourse alone; in reality, though, it's a minority for whom that is true. A 2017 study that looked at more than 1000 American women aged 18–94 found that just 18 per cent of women reached orgasm from vaginal penetration alone.[8]

It's a relatively new phenomenon, this preoccupation with the so-called vaginal orgasm. Before the eighteenth century and the Enlightenment, it was believed that for conception to occur,

it was necessary for both the man and the woman to orgasm
– at the same time. To facilitate this happening, couples were
encouraged to stimulate the clitoris directly.

After it became clear that it is not a necessary component of
reproduction, the female orgasm began to *represent* something
instead, its function examined in relation to notions about femininity and female sexuality. In the early 1900s, Sigmund Freud,
the 'father of psychoanalysis' and a man with significant and
lasting influence on Western thinking, put forward his theories
about the vaginal and clitoral orgasm, suggesting that the clitoral orgasm was sexually 'immature', the type of orgasm had by
girls and young, inexperienced women. He connected it to mental health problems, linking the clitoral orgasm to neuroticism.
A woman reached sexual maturity when she was able to orgasm
'vaginally', he suggested. A century later, his claims continue to
influence how we think and talk about sex and female orgasm.[9]

Feminists have long been vocal in disputing Freud's theories
about gender and female sexuality. When Betty Friedan wrote
*The Feminine Mystique* in 1963, a book that is credited with kick-
ing off the second wave of feminism, she dedicated a whole chapter – 'The Sexual Solipsism of Sigmund Freud' – to debunking
Freud's theories about women and their apparent inferiority.[10]

Friedan poured scorn on Freud's notion of 'penis envy',
which clearly considered women as *lacking*. Freud himself
described it like this:

> The castration-complex of the girl... is started by the
> sight of the genitals of the other sex. She immediately
> notices the difference and, it must be admitted, its signifi-
> cance. She feels herself at a great disadvantage, and often
> declares that she would like to have something like that too
> and falls victim to a penis envy, which leaves ineradicable

traces in her development and character-formation, and even in the most favourable instances, is not overcome without a great expenditure of mental energy.[11]

Friedan points out that Freud's notions about women's sexuality reflected his own preoccupations – and his own privileged, cloistered background:

> Since all of Freud's theories rested, admittedly, on his penetrating, unending psychoanalysis of himself, and since sexuality was the focus of all his theories, certain paradoxes about his own sexuality seem pertinent. His chief biographer, [Ernest] Jones, pointed out that he was, even for those times, exceptionally chaste, puritanical and moralistic. In his own life, he was relatively uninterested in sex. There was only the adoring mother of his youth, at sixteen, a romance that existed purely in fantasy with a girl named Gisele, and his engagement to Martha [his wife] at twenty-six.

It is bizarre that Freud's theories about female orgasm retained such significance in the face of scientific research and the lived experience of women, but when you consider how neatly they align with patriarchal values, it makes a little more sense. The suggestion that a vaginal orgasm is superior to a clitoral one puts a penis – or certainly a phallic object – at the centre of sex. It also prioritizes the most reliable way for a straight man to orgasm: penis-in-vagina sex.

In 1968, Anne Koedt wrote a powerful, and hugely popular, essay called 'The Myth of the Vaginal Orgasm'. She was condemnatory about Freud's role in the creation of the myth, writing:

It was Freud's feelings about women's secondary and inferior relationship to men that formed the basis for his theories on female sexuality.

It is important to emphasize that Freud did not base his theory upon a study of woman's anatomy, but rather upon his assumptions of woman as an inferior append-age to man, and her consequent social and psychological role. In their attempts to deal with the ensuing prob-lem of mass frigidity, Freudians embarked on elaborate mental gymnastics.[12]

Koedt was clear in her aims: the clitoris is the key to orgasms for women, she said, and so standard heterosexual sex should reflect this reality, or at least incorporate it. Her views on the notion of vaginal orgasm were damning: it did not exist and women who claimed it did were either confused about their own biology or were lying. 'In one case,' she writes, 'a woman pre-tended vaginal orgasm to get [a man] to leave his first wife, who admitted being vaginally frigid.'

This assertion that women were fibbing about their orgasms was widely criticized, even as the essay was lauded: who was Koedt to say that a woman's individual experience of sex and orgasm was wrong or false? Even today, that conflict remains.

Some women experience vaginal orgasm: they come through penetration alone or when they use sex toys that stimulate the walls of their vagina. But many others don't: the sex writer Karley Sciortino puts it this way: 'Sex with no clit stimula-tion just feels like I'm inserting my tampon over and over on repeat forever. It's like, "Yeah, I can *feel it*, but it doesn't feel *good*."'[13]

The most up-to-date science allows everyone to be right. We are now much more aware of the extent of the clitoris and how it interacts with the vagina during penetrative sex. We know that we can stimulate the clitoris in other places besides the super-sensitive glans. And even taking that into account, it seems there isn't just one way to orgasm. Or two or three ways. An orgasm induced by stimulating the glans of the clitoris might feel different to an orgasm that arises from vaginal stimulation, but an orgasm that results from stimulating the clitoris and the anus simultaneously might feel different again. There are countless ways to orgasm. It's not useful to categorize orgasms into clitoral or vaginal or blended categories, because if we started to categorize every orgasm, there would be an infinite number of sections and sub-sections.

Perhaps our energy would be better directed towards addressing – and closing – the 'orgasm gap', which can be defined as the difference between the number of orgasms achieved by men and women. Because, just like remuneration for work and the resulting 'pay gap', there is a huge disparity in the number of orgasms had by men and women.

In 2017, a major US study found that heterosexual women reported having fewer orgasms than any other demographic.[14] When more than 50,000 people were surveyed, 95 per cent of straight men said they usually or always orgasmed during sex, whereas only 65 per cent of straight women did. Yes, women generally find it harder to orgasm than men but when you consider that 86 per cent of lesbian women reported usually or always reaching orgasm, you can conclude that there is a specific problem occurring in straight sex. Fifty years ago, Anne Koedt wrote that 'what we must do is redefine our sexuality. We must discard the "normal" concepts of sex and create new guidelines which take into account mutual sexual enjoyment.' A quick glance at the data will tell you that as many as 35 per cent of people have failed to follow her advice.

Straight sex is still too concerned with penis-in-vagina intercourse and it continues to prioritize the man's orgasm. This feels especially true among younger couples; it was definitely the case for me when I first started having sex.

It's a point examined by Cordelia Fine, in her book *Testosterone Rex*. She writes: 'A large-scale study of thousands of female North American college students found that they had only an 11 per cent chance of experiencing an orgasm from a first casual "hookup".'[15]

This information becomes particularly pertinent when you consider how women's sexuality has been downplayed for so long, how it's been assumed that girls and women (or the respectable, well-behaved ones, anyway) are not as interested in sex outside of a committed relationship as men are.

As Fine notes: 'Some of the gap between the sexes in enthusiasm for casual sex might close if the event left men sexually frustrated the majority of the time, but women almost invariably enjoyed full sexual relief.'

It is wrong to presume that girls and women don't want sex; they just don't want *bad* or *unsatisfying* sex – and that's the type of sex they are most likely to get in a casual setting.


I think when we are young we are most at risk of believing these damaging gendered notions about sexuality: when we are young, boys' and men's sexual satisfaction is prioritized in straight relationships. As women get older, they often become more confident – about knowing what gets them off, and about asking for it.

Of course, it is not a straightforward ascent: injuries (in

the vagina, spinal cord, brain or in various other parts of the body) can affect the female orgasm, as can numerous types of medications, particularly selective serotonin reuptake inhibitors (SSRIs), which are the most commonly prescribed antidepressants. Generally, though, I believe it is true to say that women become more knowledgeable about their own bodies – and more confident with that knowledge – as they get older.

It is also true to say that some women have a better chance of achieving orgasm in a relationship, rather than during a more casual encounter. Various studies tell us various things on this issue: there is no consensus. I think there are too many amorphous elements to orgasm and desire for us ever to receive a comprehensive answer to the question: who has more orgasms – single women or those in long-term relationships? But it is something I know about myself. I find it easier to orgasm with someone I know – and perhaps love, although that's certainly not necessary. It would be wrong to interpret this as proof of my – or women's – 'more sensitive nature'. It is not that women's orgasms become more dependable, more powerful, when they are 'in love' or 'feel valued'. Rather, I think we must presume that when there is a greater level of intimacy, some women feel that they can direct their partners more readily; they can feel more comfortable in the pursuit of orgasm. They can say (in words or in unspoken communication): 'Hey, you need to touch my clitoris in exactly this way – and it really helps when you simultaneously stimulate my nipples.' Or, you know, whatever it is.

For another woman, however, the feeling of arousal that occurs from really hot casual sex, from the mystery or the implied illicitness, might be key to achieving orgasm. It's not straightforward. Various elements combine to cause orgasm – and the combination differs from person to person, from time to time, from one individual situation to the next.

The writer Roxane Gay describes it as 'the calculus of my desire'.[16] Outlining why she considers herself to be a 'bad feminist' in her book of the same name, she admits that she regularly fakes orgasms because she cannot bring herself to explain to her partners the components necessary. The way we reach orgasm can feel cringingly personal; it can feel deeply private, more private even than our naked bodies.

Gay writes:

> Sometimes—a lot of the time, honestly—I totally fake 'it' because it's easier. I am a fan of orgasms, but they take time, and in many instances I don't want to spend that time. All too often I don't really like the guy enough to explain the calculus of my desire. Then I feel guilty because the sisterhood would not approve. I'm not even sure what the sisterhood is, but the idea of a sisterhood menaces me, quietly, reminding me of how bad a feminist I am.

It's depressing to note that extra layer of shame – the guilt of letting the sisterhood down – which arrives on top of the guilt of wanting an orgasm, the guilt of not being able to orgasm, the guilt of not being able to orgasm the right way.

In any case, Gay is not unusual in admitting to faking an orgasm. It's something with which I, and many women I talk to, can identify. Sometimes, even during brilliant sex, even during sex that involves whatever kink you are into, even with a person to whom you are deeply attracted, even with direct clitoral stimulation if that's your thing, or with lots of oral if you like that, or whatever, an orgasm feels unattainable. But instead of just admitting that, instead of allowing the sex to be something that was good in and of itself, it might feel necessary to fake an orgasm, to affect an *ending*.

Perhaps Gay admits to feeling guilty about it from a feminist standpoint because she senses that by faking it, she is fibbing to protect a male ego. A 2017 American study found that heterosexual men enjoy an enhanced sense of masculinity when their partner has an orgasm during sex.[17]

It might sound counterintuitive to complain about men wanting to give women an orgasm but when it is bound up in unhelpful notions of 'manliness', it feels less about our pleasure, and more about their ego. Women don't want to feel that they *have* to writhe in pleasure, that they *have* to squirt, that they *have* to pant, that they *have* to perform as a sexual object who is in thrall to her masculine provider.

The study's authors, Sara B. Chadwick and Sari M. van Anders of the University of Michigan, put it like this:

> Women's orgasms should be experienced – when they are wanted – as a wonderful part of sexuality, not as something men give to women as an example of their prowess. Cultural ideas about masculinity push many men to feel like they need to live up to certain ideals, and this ends up being bad for sexual pleasure.[18]

It is easy to imagine that these men who feel manly about giving orgasms feel like they have discovered a 'hack' for giving a woman an orgasm, that they have discovered 'this one cool trick that is guaranteed to make her scream' while flicking through a men's magazine.

But the 'calculus of desire' cannot be hacked. It is deeply individual. What makes one woman orgasm might not work for the next; some women find it easy to orgasm, some do not.

Because of this variance, an orgasm education can never be generic. There is no applicable-to-all curriculum. But there are projects and initiatives that acknowledge this, while offering support, insight and education.

The OMGYes project, for example, offers (in its own words) 'an honest, informative, research-based approach to women's pleasure'.[19] Based on a study of 1000 American women, it identified twelve key methods of reaching orgasm, and in 2015, released a series of video tutorials, in which women carry out the techniques, touching themselves in specific ways that viewers can imitate or trial.

The result is sometimes strange: anyone who has seen standard porn will find that watching a woman masturbate in a fashion that is not designed to titillate is discombobulating. There is no moaning, no performance of pleasure. But there are genitals and breasts and nudity. For some women, it will feel superfluous, it's stuff they know already; for others, however, it could offer a breakthrough.

You can watch a woman 'layering', where she touches the skin around the clitoris rather than stimulating the exposed part. This, we are told, enables pleasure for two out of three women. You can watch women 'edging' and 'signalling' and 'staging'. You can watch women bringing themselves to orgasm in a way that is authentic and various and generous.

This one initiative will not close the orgasm gap (not everyone will be able to afford to pay to access the videos, for starters) but it is, at the very least, a high-profile acknowledgement that women masturbate, that women deserve to orgasm. Alongside projects like The Pink Protest's 2018 #GIRLSWANKTOO campaign, it reminds girls and women of the simultaneous normalcy and range of masturbation and orgasm.

It is normal, after all, to orgasm from vaginal penetration alone. It is normal, too, to orgasm only from direct clitoral stimulation. It is normal for women to ejaculate. It is normal for them not to, too. It is normal to orgasm multiple times in quick succession. It is normal to have never had an orgasm. It is normal to want to have an orgasm – and it is normal to achieve that however is easiest for you: by using the showerhead, or the strongest setting on a vibrator, or by touching yourself, or having your partner touch you in specific ways. It is normal to orgasm in your sleep. It is normal to orgasm through oral sex. It is normal to not enjoy oral sex. It is normal to rely on specific fantasies to orgasm. It is normal to feel pain after orgasm – and it is normal (it is *advisable*) to seek treatment for this. It is normal to feel teary afterwards. It is normal to feel elated, exhausted, sentimental. It is normal to enjoy sex that doesn't result in orgasm. And it is normal to not enjoy bad sex, even if you have orgasmed. It is normal to fake an orgasm. It is normal to not be able to orgasm after drinking too much alcohol or taking certain drugs. It is normal to experience unreliable and less intense orgasms at various points in your life – and it is normal to work with doctors to find out why.

There is so much that we still don't know about the female orgasm – and given how neglected the study of female sexuality has been for so long, it is hard to envisage us having all the information we crave any time soon. But by reminding ourselves of the vagaries of the female orgasm, by allowing ourselves to talk about and to investigate and to look after our own bodies, we can take a step towards a more enlightened orgasm. Education doesn't have to involve scientists or studies; it can be as simple as a frank conversation or a stolen afternoon in bed on your own or with someone you like and trust.

# CHAPTER SIX

# Appearances,
# and Looking in the Mirror

*Late last night in my bathroom…*
*After my mom went to sleep*
*I climbed up on the counter*
*And I pulled up my nightgown*
*And I* looked

*And even though*
*It was the first pussy*
*That I ever, ever saw*

*I knew* in my bones
*That no one could have*
*A pussy as perfect as mine*

*And surely a person*
*With such perfect genitals*
*Is destined for greatness*
*It's written in the stars*

Clare Barron, *Dance Nation*

Occasionally, I get a Brazilian wax. I do it around three times a year. Usually when I am going on holiday. Before I was in a long-term relationship, I think I waxed more, but my approach has always been lackadaisical.

Even though my waxes are generally associated with undressing in front of others – that is my purported reason for the expense and the pain – I find that I get a small private thrill from a wax. Not at the time, obviously, but afterwards. It feels different. Novel. More overtly sexual.

The last time I went for a wax, I was far from home, in Berlin. The woman carrying out the wax, who also seemed to own the small salon, was actually, appropriately enough, Brazilian. In her late forties, she wore a neat purple polo shirt and glasses that gave her a studious appearance.

She led me to a room, gesturing and smiling. We didn't understand each other: she spoke no English and I spoke no Portuguese; we both spoke very poor German. However, when she left the room, I knew, from previous experience, that I should take off my jeans and my knickers. I knew that I should hop up on the bed and pull a towel close to my naked crotch. It's a strange performance of privacy, this ritual that happens in waxing salons all over the world. Sure, it might feel odd to have a woman watch you undress but, in a moment, this same woman will be touching your genitals, she will be plucking hairs from your labia with tweezers.

Perhaps because of the language barrier, the fact that we could not swap niceties and anecdotes, I was more aware of the absurdity of the process than I usually am. It felt bizarre when I said 'Alles off' because I didn't know the German for 'landing strip' or 'just leave a small bit'.

It felt utterly ridiculous when she began trimming my pubic hair with a small pair of scissors. (Although, having had lots of professionals admonish me for leaving it so long between waxes, I appreciated her aura of quiet diligence. There was no tutting.)

She continued with the procedure, smoothing on the hot, luridly green wax with a spatula, then pressing it down and pulling it off, tugging out the hair.

As usual, I winced when it came to the more sensitive areas, particularly the labia – there is less hair there so it isn't as painful but the skin is so thin and, each time she pulled, I had visions of it ripping. (A tearing of the labia during a wax is not unheard of, although it is uncommon.)[1]

The strangest part of any Brazilian wax is when it's time for the professional to tackle the hair around the anus, and, lying there in Berlin, on my back, with my legs pulled to my chest and my now-bare genitalia exposed to this woman I had never met before, I thought, *What am I doing?* And why am I doing it? But then, suddenly (because the butt is always the least painful and most straightforward part), the woman was done, indicating that she was finished and I should get dressed. And it was over. And my concerns became easier to disregard.

The whole experience of paying someone to inflict pain on you by pulling your pubic hair out by the roots is undeniably bizarre – but it's also completely normalized and a fairly regular part of grooming for lots of women in the developed West. In plenty of cultures, pubic hair is seen as a symbol of fertility – some women in South Korea even have hair transplants on their vulvas, so celebrated is a thick and full bush.[2]

Generally, though, in the US and Europe the removal of pubic hair, either by waxing, shaving or using laser treatment, which has more permanent results, is pretty standard, especially for younger women. In 2016, a UK survey found that half of all women under the age of thirty-five have regular Hollywood or Brazilian waxes, removing all or most of their pubic hair.[3]

Brazilian waxing as we know it started in the late 1980s when the J Sisters salon in Manhattan began offering the service. The thinking went that it allowed women to wear a thong bikini without showing their pubic hair, but it always had connotations of sex, too. In the 1990s and early 2000s, it was generally seen as something a woman might do occasionally, especially if she was 'sexually adventurous', but now, twenty or so years later, it is a much more everyday practice. I know women who would never go longer than six weeks without a full wax. And while there were murmurs of a trend for the full-bush Brazilian (full bush but bare underneath, for people who like the sensation of bare genitals but prefer the more low-key hippie look) around 2014, the most enduringly popular wax seems to be the Hollywood, where all hair is removed.

For as long as the Brazilian bikini wax has existed there has been a simultaneous discussion about where it fits within a feminist agenda. Are waxes inherently bad for women, a consequence of living in a patriarchy that wants to deny adult female sexuality? Or should feminism encourage women to pursue sexual pleasure however they like: if a woman prefers the sensation of receiving oral sex when her vulva is hairless, why place a value judgement on that?

As far as feminist battles go, including vagina-based feminist battles, I believe there are far bigger and more pressing issues than pubic hair: eradicating period poverty, ending FGM and lobbying for better care for women who have recently given birth, for example. But I can understand how it has become a feminist touchstone – and the fact that the default vulva in modern porn is bald has a lot to do with that.

People have been removing their pubic hair for millennia – in ancient Egypt and Greece, both men and women removed their pubic hair, and most paintings of nude women depict hairless vulvas – but, for centuries, the no-hair look was not the standard for the average woman. Porn didn't revolutionize our pubic hair overnight (and it didn't do it on its own) but the general gist is that the vast majority of porn performers in film and magazines had full bushes until *Hustler* magazine printed a bald vulva, a so-called 'pink shot', in 1974. Slowly over the next two decades, pubic hair in porn disappeared and by the time Internet porn arrived, the bald vulva had become the standard. Now, pubic hair is seen as a kind of kink or fetish in porn; a preference for looking at a woman who has not shaved, waxed or lasered down there is somehow considered unusual.

The reasoning given for the baldness of most porn per-formers' genitals is that it makes it easier to see sex occur; hair blocks the view. This is connected to a reason given by some people I talk to who say they prefer a bald vulva. They like to see the genitalia clearly, they tell me, and waxing allows for that. I understand the thinking. After a wax, my genitals feel more apparent – even to me. I think of my vulva more often, because I see it more often, and so I think of sex more often.

Another regularly cited reason for preferring a sexual part-ner to have no pubic hair is that it makes giving oral sex more enjoyable – some people don't like getting stray hairs in their mouths. Perhaps connected to that preference is the notion that pubic hair is somehow unhygienic. A 2016 survey of more than 3000 American women found that 59 per cent of women who regularly remove their pubic hair do so for 'hygiene purposes'. When these same women were asked for specific situations for which they groom their pubic hair, the most common reasons were sex and holidays, but not far behind was a visit to the doc-tor's. Four in ten women said that they had groomed their hair in preparation for a doctor's appointment.[4]

The idea that pubic hair is inherently unhygienic is

fundamentally false – yes, waxing means that you are less likely to get pubic lice, but pubic lice are already very rare in the UK. Meanwhile, doctors point out that pubic hair actually performs a hygienic function, preventing bacteria from entering the vagina by trapping it, along with sweat. There is also a correlation between an increased likelihood of contracting a sexually transmitted disease (STD) and removing all of your pubic hair. A 2016 American study found that people who groomed their pubic hair daily or weekly were about three-and-a-half to four times more likely to report having an STD history.[5] There are, of course, lots of factors that influence this finding: people who remove their pubic hair tend to have more sexual partners than those who don't, but even when researchers took that and other factors like age into account, a link was found between the removal of pubic hair and STDs. The results are far from conclusive and more research is needed, but many doctors thought the findings reiterated the idea that pubic hair serves a purpose. Certainly, the correlation between grooming and STDs seems to explode the notion that pubic hair is inherently *unhygienic*.

This idea that a woman's pubic hair is somehow *dirtier* than a bald vulva goes beyond hygiene, taking in aesthetics. In 2013, the Canadian artist Petra Collins posted a picture of her crotch on Instagram. She was wearing underwear so there was no visible genitalia but pubic hair protruded from the top and sides of her green pants. The picture was removed from the social media platform, although it had violated none of the official guidelines: there was no nudity and no violence. Collins called it censorship, pointing out that it suggested a distaste for the adult female body.[6]

The incident proved just how unaccustomed we have become to images of pubic hair and to pubic hair itself – how baldness has become the norm. Recently, I was in a bar with two friends:

a man in his early thirties and a woman in her mid-twenties. We had had a few drinks and we were talking about sex, feminism, vaginas and pubic hair.

My male friend said that he preferred it when his girlfriend had a full bush. My female friend was incredulous: she couldn't quite fathom a man who didn't prefer a bald vulva. Essentially, I think that the decision to remove your pubic hair is personal – but it can be disheartening to observe how some women feel pressured to remove it. Because they want to comply with a beauty standard set by porn and Instagram. Or because they feel that their sexual partner demands it. Or because they think it's fundamentally more hygienic.

When pubic hair is removed, the genitals are obviously more visible. That can lead to an increased thrill but it can also result in a heightened sense of self-consciousness. When you can see your vulva more clearly – your labia and your clitoris – you can also see what you perceive to be *imperfections* more clearly.

Labiaplasty – surgery for reshaping or resizing the inner labia – is the fastest-growing type of plastic surgery in the world: in 2016, 45 per cent more labiaplasty procedures were carried out than in 2015, according to data gathered by the International Society of Aesthetic Plastic Surgery.[7]

Doctors in the UK have reported encountering girls as young as nine who are distraught by the appearance of their vulvas. The NHS says labiaplasty should not be carried out on girls before they turn eighteen but in 2015–16, more than 200 girls under eighteen had labiaplasty on the NHS; more than 150 of them were under fifteen.[8]

In the vast majority of cases of girls and women getting labiaplasty, there is no medical reason for the surgery. It is normal for the inner labia to be longer than the outer labia – and there is variation from woman to woman. Some girls and women will also notice how their labia change over time – the inner labia grow during adolescence and so might appear more prominent when a girl is still developing; they might appear different after vaginal childbirth.

Occasionally, a woman might experience physical discomfort if her inner labia are longer than her outer labia, especially during exercise or sex, but doctors who are seeing teenagers seeking labiaplasty report that the exaggerating of physical symptoms is not uncommon. Dr Naomi Crouch, a leading adolescent gynaecologist, has said that in her work for the NHS she has yet to see a girl who needed the operation.[9]

When you bear in mind that labiaplasty carries risks – including infection, pain during sex, scarring and lack of sensation – it seems baffling that girls and women who do not need the procedure for medical reasons are putting themselves through this.

So why the sudden upsurge? The prevalence of the bald vulva has been linked to the increase in labiaplasty, as has porn. In mainstream porn, vulvas tend to look pretty similar, with the inner labia usually sitting inside the outer labia. Some porn performers will have had labiaplasty, some will have labia that just happen to look like that, and some of the images will have been Photoshopped. Generally, porn is not presenting us with a cross-section of vulvas; instead it's showing us one type over and over again.

The fact that vaginas and vulvas are considered so private, so unknown, so taboo, allows the damaging idea that there is only one type of acceptable vulva to thrive. If you exist in a society in which nudity is unusual – and in the UK and US, public nudity is pretty rare – but porn is prevalent, you are going to grow up with a distorted view of what a vulva looks like. And where there is ignorance and insecurity, plastic surgeons will swoop.

Of course, there are surgeons carrying out labiaplasty because they feel it will benefit the comfort or sex lives of their patients – but you don't have to look too far to encounter doctors who seem preoccupied with appearances.

A Californian gynaecologist called Dr Red Alinsod has introduced a procedure that removes the inner labia completely – it's called the 'Barbie' and it creates a 'clamshell' look.[10] Like her permanently arched feet and her nipple-less breasts, Barbie's genitals are woefully unrealistic. As Peggy Orenstein points out in *Girls & Sex*, 'Barbie is (a) made of plastic and (b) *has no vagina*.'[11]

Browsing the website of another male California-based gynaecologist, Dr David Ghozland, I come across a blog that links the increased popularity of spin classes with the surge in labiaplasty. The blog suggests that women with 'excessive' and 'uneven' inner labia may find an exercise class that involves sitting on a bicycle seat uncomfortable. It goes on to connect women wearing exercise clothes to labiaplasty. 'Plastic surgeons also speculate the growing popularity of athleisure (rocking the yoga pants all day) has caused women to become more self-conscious of their nether regions,' the blog states.[12]

I envisage the women attending a Los Angeles spin class. I know that so many of them, like so many women everywhere, will have been made to feel bad about their bodies at some point. About their stomachs. Or their thighs. Or their teeth. Or their hair. Or their noses. And now, it's their vulvas. Underneath their sportswear, inside their underwear, there is another part of them that has been deemed not quite perfect. And the solution? It should be cut and clipped to fit.

Dr Jacqueline Lewis, a consultant plastic surgeon working

in London, has seen the increased demand in labiaplasty first-hand at her private clinic. She tells me that she regularly turns away potential labiaplasty clients because she does not deem surgery necessary but she will carry it out if 'they've got irritation, if it interferes with their personal hygiene or doing sport, if it's really noticeable in clothes'. Dr Lewis also points the finger at the athleisure trend, saying: 'There's the fashion now, to wear fitted clothes and leggings – you know, how a lot of people wear yogawear and sports leggings. And so the labia are more visible now.'

Increasingly visible labia have not just led to a rise in the number of women looking for labiaplasty; there has also been an upsurge in women seeking out a procedure known as a 'labial puff'. After the menopause and as a woman ages, there are likely to be changes in the appearance of the vulva, as skin becomes less elastic. A labial puff, which involves the labia being injected with hyaluronic acid or fat, aims to reverse any 'sagging'. There is never any medical indication for a labial puff but Dr Lewis says, 'I suppose you'd look better in fitted clothes and bikinis and your gym wear. You know, you would just get the cosmetic benefit and the psychological benefit and the confidence from that.'

It seems bizarre and disheartening to me that the vulva has become another body part for women to fret about and spend money on. When I was twelve and taking a first look at my vulva, I felt fearful, apprehensive, aroused, bewildered and intrigued. Completely absent, however, was any conception of the perceived *attractiveness* of my own vulva. I had been taught to compare my hair and face and hips and breasts and skin and legs and even my ears to other girls'. But my vulva? No. That was mine, a private domain and one not held to beauty standards.

Surgical treatments like labiaplasty and non-surgical treatments like labial puffs are expensive, costing thousands of pounds, and consequently they are still quite rare – but there are brands and companies aiming to attract a consumer who has less to spend. Alongside haircare and skincare, there is now vulva- and vagina-care. 'The vagina is moving into a hair-and-face space,' a trend forecaster tells me. Not so long ago, buying a product aimed at the vulva or vagina was something a person would do if she had a 'problem down there': thrush or BV, for example. (Vaginal douches and washes are actually more likely to exacerbate or even cause problems such as thrush and BV but so many consumers remain unaware of that.) Now though, there are products designed to *indulge* your vulva. There are sheet masks to 'plump' your vulva and oils to 'soften your pubic hair' (these are genuine products – I am not making this up). The new vulva- and vagina-care industry talks a lot about empowering women – and while it is true that it is refreshing to see the words 'vagina' and 'vulva' on beauty websites and it is true that it is progressive that women are being encouraged to touch and get to know their own vulvas, it is alarming that it is all in aid of selling us something we don't need.

I see a 'Moon Juice Yoni Oil' that costs £40 for a measly 30ml on one well-designed site aimed at millennials with plenty of disposable income. 'Safe to use around the vulva, this oil is great as an extra pampering step in your beauty routine,' the blurb reads. I wonder what the oil actually *does*. And that worries me – because traditionally when there hasn't been a clear need for a product, the industry has had to create one: usually by making women feel bad. The old (and still popular) 'intimate' washes and wipes and douches created a need that didn't exist by stoking fears about smell and hygiene. The new oils and masks are relying on some of those old fears while also creating a new fear that a vulva isn't fully realized, isn't fully empowered, until it has had money spent on it.

The day after I get my alles off wax in the Berlin salon, I look at my vulva, to try to understand how I feel about its *appearance*. And I feel… I don't know… nothing. I realize that my inner labia are longer than my outer labia and I notice that one side is longer than the other. But even taking in this information as I examine my body in the mirror, I feel unperturbed. I don't feel empowered. I don't feel worried. I feel nothing. I am lucky, probably, to experience this lack of concern about the appearance of my own vulva. I wish everyone could care as little as I do.

# CHAPTER SEVEN

# Periods, and What Makes Them So Awful

*It is during her periods that she feels her body most painfully as an obscure, alien thing; it is, indeed, the prey of a stubborn and foreign life that each month constructs and then tears down a cradle within it; each month all things are made ready for a child and then aborted in the crimson flow.*

Simone de Beauvoir, *The Second Sex*

*Crime scene in ur pants.*
*Ain't no man could handle that.*
*Maybe a marine.*

@SarahKSilverman, 'Menstrual Cycle Haiku', Twitter

Just after she turned eleven, my little sister got her period for the first time. It was a Sunday and we were sitting down to eat our lunch when she left the room and motioned for my mother to follow her. A short time later, my mother returned. 'She's got her period,' she said quietly. 'She's a bit upset about it.'

I started crying instantly. There is a Western trend to celebrate first periods, people even have parties, and, as a big eighteen-year-old sister, this was perhaps the tack I should have taken. I should have bounded over to my little sister who was curled up on the sofa in the next room and said, 'Congratulations!' Instead, I started weeping and when I got up from the table and went to look at her little child's face, embarrassed and scared, and her little child's body, contorted in pain, I felt even more upset.

'I'm too young,' she said. 'I don't want it.'

I tried to reassure her that plenty of girls have their periods at eleven – and I wasn't making it up: the average age for a first period is twelve, but around 13 per cent of girls are menstruating aged eleven.[1]

I said that she'd get used to it and I told her that I'd buy her strong painkillers and make her a hot water bottle once a day for seven days of each month. But I couldn't make myself feel celebratory. Because, truthfully, periods are horrible, and I didn't want my little sister – young and innocent and sweet – to have to endure the deep cramps and the stained pants and the bloated belly and the mess and the blood. She was prepared, anyway; she knew the facts. She'd grown up the youngest of three sisters and she'd been taught about menstruation. There was little that I could say to reassure her. Her sadness was, in some ways, rational.

She understood that she was at the end of childhood now and that alongside the thrill of new freedoms and new experiences would be new pains and new stigmas. It didn't help that she (accurately) associated periods with sex and fertility; this, she knew, was the end of innocence unbound by strict gender roles and the beginning of her body as a thing to be admired by men, a vessel to carry babies.

The French feminist Simone de Beauvoir acknowledged this unhappy and bloody end of girlhood in *The Second Sex*, writing:

> Previously the little girl, with a bit of self-deception, could consider herself as still a sexless being, or she could think of herself not at all; she might even dream of awakening changed into a man; but now, mothers and aunts whisper flatteringly: 'She's a big girl now'; the matron's group has won: she belongs to it. And so she is placed without recourse on the woman's side.[2]

(It is interesting to read that passage now, decades after it was written, when we are more aware of the trauma trans and non-binary teenagers endure during puberty. When a teenager who does not identify as female begins to menstruate, it can be particularly upsetting and discombobulating.)

De Beauvoir recognized that the beginning of menstruation is sometimes welcomed, with girls celebrating this new symptom of womanhood, but ultimately she came to the same sad conclusion that my sister and I arrived at:

> But the little girl is soon undeceived, for she sees that she has gained no new privileges at all, life following its usual course. The only novelty is the untidy event that is repeated each month; there are children who weep for hours when they realize that they are condemned to this fate.

De Beauvoir was writing in the 1940s, when menstruation was more of a taboo and sex education far less common, with children and teenagers sometimes completely baffled and terrified by the arrival of their periods. It was a different time. Even that Sunday when my little sister first got her period is more than fifteen years ago. So, perhaps, things are better now. Perhaps things have changed. Perhaps girls feel more prepared. Perhaps first periods are less horrible.

Well, not really – certainly not everywhere and not always. In the UK in 2017, one in four girls said that they felt unprepared for the start of their period – and one in seven did not know what was happening to them when they first began menstruating.[3] That means that around 14 per cent of girls in the UK feel scared and shocked and bewildered when they see blood in their pants for the first time. In communities and countries where sex education is less common and there is more stigma surrounding menstruation, the figures are even higher: in 2014, NGO Femme International found that 75 per cent of girls in Nairobi's Mathare Valley area had 'little idea of what menstruation was' before their first period.[4]

That absence of knowledge undoubtedly makes a first period much more traumatic; seeing unexpected blood is alarming and frightening. But even besides that, even in the best-case scenario of a girl getting her first period surrounded by a family that is supportive and encouraging, a first period can feel distressing.

But was I right to allow my sister to think that a period is horrible? And if we must say it's horrible – what makes it horrible? Is it horrible because of the biological reality of blood and pain? Or is it horrible because of the associations of womanhood and the resulting stigmas?

Let's start with the biological reality. A period occurs on Day One of a woman's monthly menstrual cycle. (Some people will have regular twenty-eight-day cycles; others will have longer or shorter cycles. Irregular cycles, where you might have a short cycle one month and a longer one the next, are especially common in adolescence or as women approach menopause. Irregular periods are also a symptom of PCOS, a condition that affects as many as one in five women.)

In the weeks prior to Day One, the endometrium – which is the mucous membrane that lines the womb – has been thickening in preparation for receiving and nourishing a fertilized egg. Most months, however, it won't receive a fertilized egg, so, on Day One, the womb begins to shed the thickened lining and expel it as a period through the vagina.

Period blood is not just blood – it comprises the thickened endometrial cells, vaginal mucus and old uterine tissue as well as blood from the arteries in the uterus. Period blood smells of blood, but also of the bacteria in your vagina. If you notice an unusually strong or unpleasant smell during your period, you should, like at any other time, see a doctor.

Period blood is often brown at the beginning or end of a period: brown blood generally means that the blood is older blood – it has had time to interact with oxygen and so it has changed from a bright red to brown. This usually indicates that it is flowing at a slower pace.

When the blood is flowing quickly, it is usually a bright red colour – generally, during a period, this means a heavier flow. It is normal for there to be clots in period blood occasionally, especially on the heaviest days. Doctors and experts don't agree on what exactly causes the clots but it is agreed that if clots are large and frequent, it is worth seeing your GP, who will refer you to a specialist.

When I have my period, I usually start out with brown blood and a light flow, progressing to deep red with occasional clots. There are days when I have vibrant red blood – like the blood from a cut – and then at the end of my period, it trails out, back to brown. Those middle days are when I worry about blood leaking, those are the days when if I don't have a menstrual cup or a pad or both, I panic. At the beginning and end of my period, the light flow of brown blood would not be likely to seep through my underwear.

It is the middle days that I find most painful, too. This hasn't always been the case; when I was younger, the first and second days of my period were the most painful. The pain was so bad that I would lie in bed, unable to move or stand, waiting to pass out in a foggy agony for a few hours at a time. I'd often get diarrhoea, too, which I have since learnt is quite common in menstruating women.

There are various types of period pain – there is period pain that is caused directly by a period and there is period pain that is caused by an underlying condition, like fibroids or endometriosis.

When I was twelve and sweating and crying and struggling with diarrhoea each month, that was, I think, the first type of period pain. This type of pain occurs when the muscular wall of the womb contracts vigorously to encourage the lining to shed. These contractions can temporarily cut off the blood supply to the womb. The blood carries oxygen, and without oxygen the tissues in your womb release chemicals that trigger pain.

While the body is releasing these pain-triggering chemicals, it also produces prostaglandins, which are chemicals that encourage the womb to contract more. It is thought that people who experience particularly bad period pain have higher levels of prostaglandins. Prostaglandins are also responsible for the diarrhoea and nausea some of us get around our period, as when prostaglandins are sent to the womb, they may make it to the nearby bowel, which will contract, too.[5]

When I was a young teenager, I was prescribed hormonal contraception as a means of minimizing the period pain I was experiencing and today, two decades on, that is still the most effective way to treat the problem for those living in the developed world with easy access to contraception. When taking the contraceptive pill or using other hormonal contraception like an intrauterine system (IUS), most people will experience much lighter and less painful bleeding around the time of their period. Some people will find that using hormonal contraception means that they stop bleeding completely or only bleed for a day or two each month.

For years, I relied on hormonal contraception but eventually – because, like many women, I was worried that it affected my mood – I stopped and I found that the period pain was much less intense in my twenties than it had been in my teens.

This is considered normal – period pain that doesn't have an underlying cause often gets better with age, although periods vary throughout our lives and differ from person to person. Some women report that the pain significantly decreases after having children. Others find their periods get heavier and more painful after pregnancy and childbirth.

In my thirties, I began to get period pain again, the type that wakes me up in the middle of the night with its intensity. It almost makes me laugh, I feel giddy with the pain, hot and light in my head, as the deep agony pulses through my lower abdomen, spreading to my legs, unsteadying them.

I find that if I get on all fours and pull my stomach in towards my spine, there is a sense of relief. I also like to sit on the loo with my pants pulled down, bent over, pulling my elbows into myself. Hot water bottles help, too, almost because the sensation of the heat on my skin is a distraction.

I have been to the doctor about this new period pain and I have had ultrasounds and vaginal exams. It might be fibroids, the doctors have said, but without conviction or certainty. There are fibroids present in my womb but they can't be sure if those are big enough to be causing the pain. Taking hormonal contraception is not an option for me at this stage of my life as I am hoping to get pregnant and, instead, I have been prescribed tranexamic acid, which reduces blood loss, and mefenamic acid, which is a nonsteroidal anti-inflammatory drug (NSAID) and prohibits prostaglandins. When I take the tranexamic acid and the mefenamic acid alongside co-codamol tablets I buy over the counter, I find that I can usually bear the pain, although some months it still causes me to miss work or dates with friends.

I've had my period since I was twelve and I'll probably have it for around another fifteen years. So let's say I menstruate once a month for thirty-seven years and I usually have my period for five days each month – that's sixty days a year multiplied by thirty-seven years, so that's 2200 days. Or around six years of bleeding over a lifetime.

That's a lot – but if I were to calculate *all* the time that my period affects me, I'd have to factor in premenstrual syndrome (PMS), too. I don't get PMS every month but I get it a lot; let's round it out at one day a month for thirty-seven years, bearing in mind that some months I'll have five days of PMS, other months nothing. That's a year and a half of PMS over a lifetime.

Sometimes it's not so bad, just some light bloating. Other months, it descends as an unsettled depression and a strange feeling in my legs. On those months, tears and anger come scarily easily. And I'm not alone – most women experience at least some symptoms of PMS and 5–8 per cent of women get premenstrual dysphoric disorder (PMDD). PMDD leads to more extreme feelings of depression, anxiety and lethargy. And while there are suggestions that PMS and PMDD are not biological but actually cultural or social, I – and plenty of scientists and academics – would refute that charge.

So, there we are, that's the biology of my period. Some people will have less severe symptoms and some will struggle more – but that's my biological lot. And in a lot of ways, it's horrible.

Intensifying all that messy pain is the stigma of a period.

Roughly half of all women in the world are of reproductive age so around a quarter of the world's population – including trans men and non-binary people – gets a period every month. And yet, still, it feels like it's something almost *secret*, a private suffering to be endured with quiet stoicism by each individual. It is still too rare for periods, and their symptoms, to be spoken of openly – in workplaces, in schools, in our culture.

For years, I worked in an office that was staffed only by women and non-binary people: it was the kind of place where we would post 'Does anyone have any tampons?' on Slack and shout 'We're synched' if we got our periods at the same time. (The synching of periods for women who live or work or spend a lot of time together has pretty much been scientifically disproven but sometimes it is still fun to pretend it exists.) When a male CEO was appointed, he began making changes and at one stage, he said, 'There's going to be a lot less period talk around here.' Was he joking? We weren't sure. But I felt less comfortable making a soothing hot water bottle for myself or my menstruating colleagues after that.

Period leave – legalized time off for employees experiencing menstrual cramps – is actually a reality for some, but it's not always an uncomplicated advantage. Since 1947, Japanese women have been entitled to menstrual leave but very few women avail of it – either because they do not know they are entitled to it or they fear they will be stigmatized or sexually harassed if they do take it.[6]

There have been murmurs about the introduction of legalized time off for employees experiencing menstrual cramps in the UK, and some companies have been leading the way and implementing period leave policies of their own. In 2016, a Bristol company called Coexist, which manages arts spaces in the city, made headlines with its period leave policy. Bex Baxter, the director of Coexist, started thinking about the idea of period leave in 2015 and when, in March 2016, she organized a seminar inviting 100 businesses to learn about the power of the menstrual cycle as an asset to organizations, it led, she tells me, 'to the international media going wild'. The story was picked up in all the major papers and news organizations, prompting both consternation and support. It was another year before the policy could be implemented: there were six months of staff consultations followed by a six-month-long pilot scheme.

When I speak to Baxter, Coexist's period policy has been in place for just over a year. So, how exactly does it work, I ask. Baxter explains:

> In every department, the menstruators have got their menstrual charts on the wall, so people know when they're having their period, it's talked about really openly. It's a normal conversation – in check-ins before meetings, people go round and say how they are and people say I'm on day three, or I'm feeling like this because of my period.

And what if people don't want to tell their colleagues they're feeling tetchy or tired, what if they don't want to draw attention to their own bodies, their own biology, their own pain, at work? 'It's an opt-in opt-out policy,' says Baxter. 'Some women don't suffer, and they don't feel the need to have it. Some women don't suffer, but they recognize that at the time of menstruation, you may not be tired but you need to go slower, because then the rest of your day works properly.'

A year in, Baxter considers the scheme a success but says she prefers the term 'menstrual flexi-time policy' to 'period leave':

A lot of women are terrified – that's why they don't take up these policies. They think it will make them less employable, even if it's offered. But what we found was that if women could take time out and put it back in, or if there are contingency plans that take care of that, it's a more beneficial thing.

Baxter says she considers the 'crude productivity financial side' of menstrual policies but it's not hard to imagine other leaders, with different priorities, considering the productivity of employees and deciding there should be less period chat – and fewer period-related sick days.

Sally Rooney's 2017 novel *Conversations with Friends* is a rare example of a piece of art that actually engages with the reality of living with menstruation. The protagonist and narrator Frances struggles with acute period pain. Her agony turns out to be related to endometriosis but the descriptions of the monthly pains resonated with me, as someone who has lain on bathroom tiles, willing hours and days away.

A particular passage stays with me:

I hit my forehead against the side of the bath to distract myself from the pain in my pelvis. It was a hot pain, like all my insides were contracting into one little knot... Eventually it got light outside. Bobbi woke up and came in to help me onto the couch in the living room. She made

me a cup of peppermint tea and I sat slouched holding
the cup against my T-shirt, just above my pubic bone,
until it started to scald me.[7]

The way the character manufactures other pain to distract from
the period pain is a tactic I identify with, but, besides the specifics, this description of period pain felt powerful to me simply
because it was an acknowledgement of something I experience.
And I have very rarely had that experience acknowledged in novels or in films or in TV shows.

Period pain is perhaps not dramatic – the regularity of it as
well as the easily explained cause means that, most of the time,
a narrative involving period pain will not feature twists and
turns and big reveals. But to read about it in a novel felt important to me. I felt comforted and moved and interested. When
I interviewed Rooney, I asked her about the representation of
menstruation in *Conversations with Friends* and its absence in
the majority of literature. She said: 'I do sometimes think about
how, if an alien race were to review the history of English literature, they would not know that women menstruate even though
we do it quite a lot. But you never encounter it – it's not, like,
ever mentioned in a Victorian novel.'[8]

We deny periods, we gloss over periods, we hide periods. We
ignore them, suffer through them, tampons stuffed up sleeves
and euphemisms deployed. Of course, if cisgender men got
periods things would probably be different. It's a point made
in Gloria Steinem's 1978 *Ms* magazine essay, 'If Men Could
Menstruate':

So what would happen if suddenly, magically, men could
menstruate and women could not?
    Men would brag about how long and how much...

Sanitary supplies would be federally funded and free...

Street guys would invent slang ('He's a three-pad man') and 'give fives' on the corner with some exchange like 'Man, you lookin' good.'

'Yeah, man, I'm on the rag!'

TV shows would treat the subject openly.[9]

What Steinem was saying then, and what I am saying now, is that yes, periods are biologically horrible. But the fact that we live in a society in which the most dominant people do not get periods means that they are more horrible than they have to be due to the shame and secrecy that surrounds them.

The period stigma has been around for thousands of years. The word 'taboo' is even thought to derive from the Polynesian word 'tupua', which means menstruation.[10]

It was around when I was a teenager – I remember a boy telling me that his friend had a horse that would buck violently when mounted by a girl who was menstruating. This boy's disgust for girls and their blood was evident – he commended the horse on his instincts.

It was around in Roman times, too, when Pliny the Elder wrote *Natural History*, a work that is considered to be the first encyclopaedia and informed thinking on science for centuries afterwards. On periods, he was clear: they were an abomination, potentially responsible for all manner of evil and misfortune.

He wrote:

Contact with the monthly flux of women turns new wine sour, makes crops wither, kills grafts, dries seeds in gardens, causes the fruit of trees to fall off, dims the bright surface of mirrors, dulls the edge of steel and the gleam of ivory, kills bees, rusts iron and bronze, and causes a horrible smell to fill the air. Dogs who taste the blood become mad, and their bite becomes poisonous as in rabies.[11]

(It's pretty clear to me now that the teenage boy who boasted that his friend's misogynist horse hated menstruation had probably, actually been influenced by Pliny the Elder, 2000 years on.)

In some Nepalese communities, there is still a belief – tied to ancient Hindu culture – that menstruating women are toxic, capable of contaminating food and killing crops. The Nepalese tradition of chhaupadi declares that menstruating girls and women should be banished to huts for the duration of their periods. Women have faced grave danger obeying this tradition – in 2017, a woman died having been bitten by a poisonous snake while in exile and there have been reports of women being raped while staying in these isolated locations. In 2017, the Nepalese government made it illegal to force a woman to obey chhaupadi but it continues to be practised. In January 2018, a twenty-two-year-old woman called Gauri Kumari Bayak died from asphyxiation in a rural part of Nepal: she had started a fire to keep herself warm while banished to a hut.[12]

In almost every faith, there is a squeamishness around periods. A 2018 report found that in both Catholic and Protestant schools in Northern Ireland, the use of tampons was considered contentious, as inserting them into the vagina was associated with sexual maturity. Similarly, there is sometimes a reluctance to recommend or prescribe hormonal contraception to teenagers suffering with period pain because of its associations with sex.[13]

Muslim girls and women are not supposed to pray or fast during their periods – which can lead to self-consciousness for young people who are menstruating. By not praying or fasting, they are *announcing* they have their period – and, at twelve or thirteen, that can feel embarrassing. Sex during menstruation is also forbidden.

In the orthodox Jewish community, girls and women become a niddah while menstruating and are considered to be impure during this time. Sex is not allowed during niddah and only after the period has ended and a ritual bath called a mikvah has been taken, can a woman be considered pure again.

When poverty – a state often seen as shameful and taboo – combines with periods, the stigma and the difficulties can intensify. In 2017, period poverty became front-page news in the UK when a charity in Leeds revealed that girls were missing school because they couldn't afford sanitary towels and tampons. Girls were stuffing their pants with socks and toilet paper, reluctant or frightened to ask parents who were already struggling with household budgets to fork out a tenner a month for pads and tampons.[14]

In 2015, a study conducted in Kenya found that 10 per cent of the fifteen-year-old girls that the researchers questioned had 'had sex for money' so that they could afford sanitary towels. [15] The same study revealed that 25 per cent of women in the rural Kenyan community where the study took place were relying on makeshift items – newspaper, discarded cloths, leaves – when they were menstruating. When girls and women are forced to resort to improvised sanitary products, there can be real and serious consequences, with the material spreading dirt and bacteria, resulting in urinary and reproductive tract infections.

All over the world, people who menstruate face avoidable distress and discrimination. In US prisons, tampons and sanitary towels are used as bargaining chips, with inmates being humiliated and facing health crises when access is limited.[16]

In Odisha, a state in eastern India, 20 per cent of girls (and, tellingly, 35 per cent of disabled girls) don't go to school while they have their period, missing hours and days and weeks and months of education.[17]

Periods are painful and messy because of biology. And cultural, social, religious and economic forces make them worse.

But is there hope? I will continue to get my period every month until I go through the menopause, perhaps stopping for pregnancy and periods of breastfeeding. So, you know, only roughly 20,000 more hours of bleeding left. Will those hours take place in a world that is more understanding of periods? And I don't just mean *my* world – I am a white, privileged woman who works from home and can easily afford tampons and sanitary towels and expensive period-proof underwear from brands like THINX.

What I mean is: will *the world* become more understanding of periods? Will life improve for the almost two billion people who menstruate?

There are reasons to be hopeful. Several international media outlets declared 2015 as the 'year of the period', with frank conversations about menstruation taking place on websites and the radio, in magazines and newspapers.

It began in January of that year with the British tennis player Heather Watson remarking that 'girl things' had contributed to her losing a match at the Australian Open. Of course, periods are likely to affect sportswomen but the subject has been largely overlooked – both in terms of sports science research, and coverage and analysis.[18]

In March 2015, Rupi Kaur, the bestselling poet who is followed by millions on Instagram, challenged the social media platform when it removed a picture she had posted of herself with period blood on her pants. That summer, Kiran Gandhi ran the London Marathon while free-bleeding, making headlines and vowing to stand up to oppressive shaming. Three months later, two activists protested the tampon tax by free-bleeding outside the UK Houses of Parliament, their tracksuit bottoms stained red, their point powerfully made.

When periods are discussed with honesty and compassion in our culture and media, we see real and significant results. In the 2016 film, *I, Daniel Blake*, a heartbreaking scene showed a woman stealing a pack of sanitary towels from a supermarket. That moment – that fear and desperation that flicker in actor Hayley Squires's face – led to an increased awareness of period poverty and a surge in donations of menstrual products to food banks and charities.[19]

In the last few years there have been major wins for activists: at the time of writing, the tampon tax – the levy placed on menstrual products because they are bafflingly deemed as 'luxuries' – remains in place in the UK (due mainly to complicated EU law) but the government now uses the money the tax generates to fund women's projects and charities, including initiatives to fight period poverty.[20] Tesco, meanwhile, announced in 2017 that it would cover the cost of the 5 per cent tax for consumers, having reduced prices.[21] In 2018, Liverpool Football Club committed to help fight period poverty by providing free sanitary towels and tampons at its stadium, Anfield.[22]

And that blue liquid that has been a symbol of period squeamishness in advertising for decades now? Well, it – and its close friend, the leaping, laughing menstruating woman – is beginning to feel more than a little ridiculous. In 2017, the UK sanitary towel brand Bodyform (which is owned by Swedish company Essity, an operation making sanitary towels under various brands) released an advert that showed period blood. It was there just for a flash, dripping down a woman's leg in the shower. The move felt revolutionary and useful and commendable – but it's worth considering the big corporations' involvement in perpetuating period stigma in the first place.

Disposable sanitary towels were introduced around the time of World War One; up until that point most women in the US and Europe had been using cotton fabric that they washed at the end of each day, and reused. In 1914, a company called Kimberly-Clark developed a substitute for cotton – made from wood pulp, they called it Cellucotton. During the war, it became a substitute for cotton surgical dressings and Red Cross nurses quickly realized that it was also a useful material to use when menstruating. After the war, Kimberly-Clark bought back the surplus Cellucotton from the American military and began producing sanitary towels using Cellucotton and gauze. They called them Kotex and they went on sale in 1920. Tampax, the world's most famous tampon brand, was founded in the US in 1931 and enjoyed a surge in popularity after linking the product to women's labour participation during World War Two.

From the beginning, the language used in sanitary towel and tampon advertising was designed to shame and horrify. 'Women, end accident panic!' one advert for sanitary towels from 1935 commands.[23] These new products relied on the already present sense that period blood was so much more heinous, more poisonous, more embarrassing than other regular bodily fluids, like a runny nose or even urine.

It is estimated that by 2022, the global feminine hygiene industry will be worth as much as $43 billion[24] – the industry is growing as women across the developing world gain increased purchasing power. The big corporations have a guaranteed market – the billions of us who menstruate – and it is difficult not to detect a degree of greed and arrogance in the face of our dependency.

There are some big questions that this huge industry must answer. Where is the joined-up strategy to tackle period poverty across the developing and developed world? Why is the continuation of shame and stigma still considered a sensible marketing strategy? And perhaps, most pressing of all, what about the environment?

Certain brands of sanitary towels contain up to 90 per cent plastic, which is estimated to take up to 800 years to decompose.[25] Particular types of tampons come with unnecessary plastic applicators (I admit that until recently, it was these tampons I favoured – they are the least uncomfortable to insert). The use of tampons and sanitary towels creates 200,000 tonnes of waste each year, in the UK alone.[26] In 2010, a UK beach clean found an average of twenty-three sanitary pads and nine tampon applicators per kilometre of British coastline.[27]

We *are* seeing more environmentally friendly types of tampons and sanitary towels arriving on the market courtesy of smaller, more socially responsible companies, but the big brands are still overwhelmingly popular. It seems obvious that anyone who says they care about the environment should embrace, or at least *try*, period products that don't create waste – menstrual cups and period-proof underwear (pants that absorb blood).

Menstrual cups – reusable, funnel-shaped devices that collect blood in the vagina – have been around for nearly 200 years but it wasn't until they were manufactured using silicone that they became comfortable enough to go mainstream. The fact that they can be used again and again for years makes them crucial in the fight against both period poverty and unnecessary waste. There is perhaps still a squeamishness surrounding them – they do require a more *involved* approach than tampons or sanitary towels. There will be blood on your hands; your fingers will be inside your own vagina; you will have to pour the blood that collects in the cup down the toilet; you will have to wash the cup out, watching the pink water swirl down the drain – and they are not for everyone: people with certain disabilities might find some models difficult to manoeuvre and younger girls are likely to find them intimidating. In countries where women have limited access to water and toilets, they will not be practical. But plenty of people, including myself, find them comfortable (honestly, I forget I'm wearing them in a way I never did with tampons), reliable and cost-effective.

Modern women have more periods than women at any other point in history: until the twentieth century, women spent a lot of their adult life either pregnant or breastfeeding – states that halt menstruation. They also tended to start menopause – and stop menstruating – earlier. So, along with the ongoing and cumulative work of feminism, it perhaps makes sense that we are, at the beginning of the twenty-first century, reflecting on the pain and the shaming and the practicalities of periods in such an invigorated way.

And so I find myself asking: would I cry now? Would the sight of my eleven-year-old sister, curled up on the sofa, still upset me?

And would I cry in the future? Are periods getting better? And will they be even better in ten, twenty, 100 years' time?

We are tackling the stigma – slowly, certainly, and starting from a point of heinous discrimination in some cultures, yes. But we are challenging the shame. And when we do that, we are able to make a difference to the experience of having a period. As girls and women continue to make gains towards a more equal world, we are likely to see more women and people who have periods in positions of power – and if more of the scientists and researchers and inventors and legislators and CEOs have experienced menstruation, that will have an obvious impact on pain management solutions, period products, period leave policies and societal attitudes. When there is an increased openness about periods, we will see more work done to counteract their basic biological awfulness.

# CHAPTER EIGHT

# Pain, As It
# Applies to Women

*A lot of people spend their lives in pain, often because our upbringing or gender or religion or self-esteem decrees that we deserve to suffer through it, that we aren't entitled to feel good – perhaps women more than most.*

Jami Attenberg, 'Letter of Recommendation: Hysterectomies', *The New York Times Magazine* (2018)

When I began bleeding from my vagina at times when I wasn't menstruating, I went to the doctor. Not straight away, because I thought it was nothing or I thought it was normal or I thought that I couldn't afford to take an afternoon off work. But after six months or so, I went to the doctor. They tested for STDs but I didn't have any. A cervical smear showed nothing unusual. An ultrasound indicated that I had some uterine fibroids, but the sonographer said they were unlikely to be the cause of the bleeding. After a year or so of the irregular, unexplained bleeding, I was sent to my local hospital in east London for a hysteroscopy.

A hysteroscopy involves a doctor taking a tube that gushes water and has a camera attached to its tip, and inserting it into your vagina. The tube is then pushed through your vagina, through your dilated cervix and into your womb. The images that the camera picks up are relayed to a monitor near your head.

The doctor performing my hysteroscopy, one of six medical professionals in the room, seemed kind and considerate. Before I was taken to the operating theatre, he visited me on the ward and asked me if I had taken any painkillers. I told him that I had taken two co-codamol tablets and he told me that a nurse would bring me two ibuprofen tablets. After the hysteroscopy got underway, he kept asking questions like, 'Does that feel OK?' and 'Do you want me to stop?' But those questions were hard to answer – because I wanted to scream, 'No, I'm not OK' and 'Yes, please, please, stop.' Instead, though, I said, 'It's really, really painful. But whatever you think.' He was the expert. It felt as though I was going to pass out from the waves of pain breaking through my body but I figured that he knew better than me. Surely, he would know if the pain was too much, too extreme.

At one point, he gently asked if I would like to take a look at my uterus on the monitor. I thought that I would be interested – when I had the ultrasound, I peeked at the screen and I've never been squeamish about blood. But when I turned my head and was faced with a live feed of my own womb, all white and red and empty and bloody, I panicked. It felt obscene to be looking at my insides like that. And so for the rest of the procedure, I kept my eyes fixed on the ceiling.

When the pain became so bad I was crying and saying, 'Actually no, I cannot cope with this pain, please help me', the doctor gave me a little break and administered a local anaesthetic. Once he had injected me with anaesthetic, the hysteroscopy was painless. It was uncomfortable and strange but the pain had stopped.

After it was finished, the doctor told me that he thought I was fine. He confirmed that I had uterine fibroids and he said that I had a tilted uterus, but he told me there was nothing to worry about. A nurse gave me a discharge letter. It noted that I was healthy but a 'patient particularly sensitive to pain'. This jarred with my perception of myself – but there it was, in black and white.

I thought back to the pain I had endured when I was hit by a car when I was nineteen, the way the doctors had had to pull glass out of my face and legs. I remembered the sessions of physiotherapy after the car accident, the agony I'd experienced then. And I thought, *Huh, all that must not have been very painful after all. Because here I am, a woman with a letter printed by a doctor that says I am 'particularly sensitive to pain'.*

I felt grateful after the hysteroscopy – the doctor had ruled out some of the most serious potential causes of the bleeding and as a person born outside the UK, I am constantly amazed and impressed by the UK's NHS. 'It's FREE,' I shout down the phone to my Irish family whenever we discuss British healthcare in any terms.

It was only months later, when I read how hysteroscopies are usually carried out under a *general* anaesthetic in the US, that I thought, *Why did it take him so long to give me a local anaesthetic? Why did he watch me as tears rolled down my cheeks? Why did he think it was OK for me to suffer?*

I came across the US hysteroscopy description in a memoir called *An Excellent Choice: Panic and joy on my solo trip to motherhood* by the journalist and author Emma Brockes. As a Brit in New York, Brockes is interested in the differences between the UK and US healthcare systems – particularly as they pertain to fertility and childbearing. Having been told that she needed a hysteroscopy in New York, Brockes consulted both the UK and US guidelines: the Royal College of Obstetricians and Gynaecologists in the UK recommended a local anaesthetic; her New York doctor would only carry out the procedure under a general anaesthetic. Brockes notes: 'It is hard not to laugh at this, the difference in the two cultures' idea of pain management. In Britain, whether it hurts or not, it is assumed you will take it on the chin and be grateful that anyone bothered with you in the first place.'[1]

As I read that passage, I felt vindicated. I am not a person 'particularly sensitive to pain'; I am just a person who was subjected to extreme pain and expected to muddle through on some over-the-counter painkillers. And it seemed clear to me: the doctor had been nice but he had also been patronizing and dismissive.

I had lain there, with my feet in stirrups, my legs spread far apart, my genitals exposed to six people, my body convulsing in agony – and it had taken the doctor too long, way too long, to take my pain seriously and put me out of my misery by administering an anaesthetic.

And yes, there are matters of cost, there are matters of safety, I understand that, but still it felt obscene. It feels obscene to remember it, even now. The doctor took a hysteroscope and he put it in my vagina and he dilated my cervix and he filled me full of water and he watched and he listened as I cried and said, 'I am in so much pain.' And he thought that all I needed was some co-codamol and two ibuprofen tablets.

The doctor misunderstood how much pain I was experiencing. He *underestimated* how much pain I was experiencing.

*

124

The sensation of having pain misunderstood and underestimated is one familiar to most women. 'You should do some exercise if your period is painful,' a person might say to a girl and the girl will laugh bitterly – but only after she has passed out on the cold tiles in the family bathroom because the pain that accompanies her period is so intense, so unbearable, so incompatible with exercise.

Perhaps because we get periods – and periods are excruciating for so many of us – there is a sense that to be a woman involves pain, that it involves putting up with pain. A period won't kill you – there is no great medical investigation to be carried out, no mystery to unravel. Period pain is to be expected, to be endured, to be borne – with discretion and even good cheer.

In her essay, 'Grand Unified Theory of Female Pain', Leslie Jamison considers how pain has been woven into the meaning of womanhood:

> The old Greek Menander once said: '*Woman is a pain that never goes away.*' He probably just meant women were trouble. But his words work sideways to summon the possibility that being a woman *requires* being in pain; that pain is the unending glue and a prerequisite of female consciousness.[2]

We bleed each month – and that is normal. We are in pain each month – and that is normal. We give birth to a baby, sweating, wailing, stretching, tearing – and that is normal.

Even when our pain is abnormal, it is often misunderstood or minimized. Women's pain is consistently taken less seriously than men's – we know this anecdotally and from academic research.

Women wait longer for treatment in A&E departments than men, according to studies and data from Europe and the US.[3] And when women do see a doctor, they are more likely than men to receive prescriptions for sedatives – rather than pain medication.[4] It is, it seems, a more urgent priority to calm a woman than it is to treat the pain that is causing her distress in the first place. And that is a dangerous strategy, meaning that diagnoses might be missed or delayed. Generally, women's response to pain is more likely to be considered by healthcare professionals as 'emotional, psychogenic, hysterical or oversensitive'.[5]

There are, it seems true to say, differences between how men and women experience pain. There is evidence to suggest that women may engage in pain-related catastrophizing more than men.[6] And it is thought that women experience pain differently depending on where they are in their menstrual cycle – oestrogen alters the perception of pain and the response to painkillers.[7]

However, it is impossible to get a clear and detailed overview of how women react differently to pain and pain medication because we simply don't have the data. Women have been woefully neglected in studies on pain: most of our understanding of ailments – most of our medical evidence – comes from the perspective of men; it is overwhelmingly based on studies of men, carried out by men.

The fact that women have been so overlooked in studies about pain seems particularly remiss given that there is evidence to suggest that women are more likely to suffer from a chronic pain condition, which is defined as pain that lasts longer than twelve weeks despite medication and treatment.[8] Endometriosis means living with chronic pain. Vulvodynia means living with chronic pain. Both conditions involve the sexual and reproductive organs, too, and so they seem to exist surrounded by whispers, doubts, misgivings.

A pain that doesn't go away, that can't be easily vanquished; a pain that only affects women, that is linked to our womanly biology – that is a pain that is undermined and minimized and misunderstood.

In 2017, the National Institute for Health and Care Excellence (NICE) deemed it necessary to tell NHS doctors that they must 'listen to women' who presented with symptoms of endometriosis. If women present with symptoms including continuing pelvic pain, severe period pain or pain during sex, or if they suffer from infertility, endometriosis must not be ruled out, NICE counselled.[9]

It seems like appallingly obvious and overdue advice but, when you consider that it takes an average of seven to eight years to get an endometriosis diagnosis, it becomes clear that it was necessary.

Endometriosis is a condition in which tissue that is similar to the lining of the womb, the endometrium, grows outside the womb – in the fallopian tubes, the ovaries, the bladder and the bowel, for example. Each month, when pregnancy hasn't occurred, the tissue gets the signal to bleed. Endometriosis is thought to affect one in ten women of reproductive age and delayed diagnosis is a significant problem, leading to women experiencing years of pain and distress. The pain can be so extreme that women miss and lose work or see their social and sex lives contract. The pain can lead to depression and anxiety. If endometriosis is left untreated, it can get worse, organs can become fused; ultimately it can cause infertility. Endometriosis can wreck women's lives – and too many women are forced to wait too, too long before receiving treatment or care.

It is a condition that is difficult to diagnose. The symptoms vary and the only way to tell for sure that a person has endometriosis is a laparoscopy – keyhole surgery carried out under general anaesthetic. But beyond those practical concerns, there are hazier, more troubling reasons for the slow diagnoses.

When girls and women are told that womanhood is pain, they might just attempt to suffer through the symptoms of endometriosis, the excessive bleeding and the cramps.

When girls and women are told that sex is more about pleasing their partner than having an orgasm or even a good time, they might just write off the pain they experience during intercourse.

When girls and women are told that vaginas are embarrassing or private or something to be squeamish about, they might just not go to the doctor, for a few months, or for a year, or for longer.

And even if they do go to the doctor, they might be fobbed off with unhelpful advice like, 'It will go away when you get pregnant' or 'It's normal to experience bad period pain' or 'You might have IBS – why don't you try cutting out garlic and onions?'

And even if they encounter a sympathetic, knowledgeable doctor, they might come up against a warren of cul-de-sacs, dead ends about how to treat and manage the disease. More research into endometriosis is necessary, much more, especially as some leading experts believe that the disease may be getting more aggressive,[10] with some evidence linking the hormone-disrupting chemicals, phthalates and DDE – found in plastics, pesticides, shampoos, soaps, sanitary products, the list goes on and on – to endometriosis.[11]

There is no cure for endometriosis. And treatment – and access to treatment – will vary depending on where in the world you live (endometriosis is not even recognized in some countries), what kind of healthcare or medical insurance you have and the individual doctors and specialists you encounter.

In the UK, those suffering with endometriosis can alleviate symptoms with pain relief – heat packs, physiotherapy, painkillers or Transcutaneous Electrical Nerve Stimulator (TENS) machines, which are small machines with electrodes that attach to the skin and send electrical pulses into the body. Some women are prescribed the contraceptive pill or other hormonal treatments to suppress the production of oestrogen and progesterone, and that can be an effective way of treating the disease – the endometrium-like tissue won't bleed each month when ovulation and menstruation is halted.

In some cases, surgery is necessary. Deposits of the endometrium-like tissue can be excised (cut out) or destroyed (by laser or heat) during a diagnostic laparoscopy, but if the endometriosis is more severe and there are more organs involved (the bowel or bladder, for example), more complex surgery, involving a multi-disciplinary team, is needed. In rare cases, when the endometriosis has not responded to other treatments, radical surgery might be necessary. This might involve a hysterectomy (the removal of the womb) or a single or bilateral oophorectomy (the removal of one or both of the ovaries). Both surgeries are irreversible and come with significant consequences (pregnancy is no longer possible; a bilateral oophorectomy will prompt an immediate menopause), but some women suffering from endometriosis will weigh up the advantages and disadvantages and make that decision. They will make that decision knowing that radical surgery might not halt their pain, might not cure their endometriosis.

When Lena Dunham wrote an essay about having a hysterectomy at thirty-one to treat her endometriosis, she addressed the horrible, almost impossible choice:

I know it as intensely as I know I want a baby: that something is wrong with my uterus. I can feel it, deeply specific yet unverified, despite so many tests and so much medical dialogue. I just sense that the uterus I have been given is defective.[12]

A year after the hysterectomy, doctors removed Dunham's left ovary, which was encased in scar tissue and had attached to her bowel. Writing about the single oophorectomy on Instagram, she discussed the complicated nature of treatment for endometriosis:

> A lot of people commented on my last post about being too sick to finish promoting my show by saying my hysterectomy should have fixed it (I mean *should* is a weird one). That I should get acupuncture and take supplements (I do). That I should see a therapist because it's clearly psychological (year 25 of therapy, y'all. These are the fruits!) But a big lesson I've learned in all of this is that health, like most stuff, isn't linear.[13]

Alongside her words was a photograph showing Dunham lying on a hospital bed, her mesh pants pulled down and her hospital smock pulled up, to reveal a wound near her belly button. Dunham has created a career from chronicling women's pain – from break-ups and bad internships to abortions and bad sex – and in that Instagram post, she showed us her endometriosis pain. It was there to offer hope; to help to educate. But by posting it, she no doubt implicitly understood that it would be picked apart and undermined, too.

It seems particularly female, this presentation of pain. It seems that women are forced to show us their pain, forced to say, *Please believe me*, as they expose their wounds. But the benefits of women displaying their pain cannot be underestimated.

I only became aware of endometriosis after Hilary Mantel presented her pain, showed it to us all, so that we could understand it and learn from it, in a 2004 newspaper article.

Mantel has had endometriosis since she was eleven, and when she was in her late twenties, she had radical surgery, with doctors removing her womb, ovaries and parts of her bladder and bowel. Mantel possesses a rare mastery of words and so when she presents her pain – the pain of the constant bleeding, the pain of the infertility, the pain of the pain coming back even after radical surgery, the pain of the drug treatments that cause weight gain – it is wrenching and visceral. 'Fatigue and intermittent pain are still my companions,' she tells us. 'My soul rattles around in its capacious house, and dwells on the life I might have had…'[14]

The pain of endometriosis is compounded, made even more tortuous, when the pain is not believed, understood or acknowledged. And in the 1970s and 1980s, when Mantel was first seeking treatment, there was widespread scepticism. She writes:

> Myths about the condition had made their way into the textbooks. Endometriosis patients were 'anxious perfectionists', white, middle-class career women in their 30s. The truth was, it was these well-educated nags who were getting a correct diagnosis.

Even decades on, I don't think it's wrong to suspect that it is 'well-educated nags' who can more quickly access diagnoses, treatment and care. Sometimes – and especially with conditions relating to the vagina, the vulva and the reproductive organs – it feels like a woman must meticulously build her case; she must make herself believable, convincing. She must describe her pain, but not seem hysterical. She must record her symptoms, but not seem paranoid.

'White, middle-class career women in their 30s' possess more privilege than women of colour or trans people or other minorities, and are, I would guess, more likely to be believed and listened to.

There isn't much data (how many times must I type 'more research is needed' during the course of writing this book?) about the discrepancy in how the pain of white women and women of colour is treated, but studies point to the possibility of racial bias. The subject has been given more attention in the US, where a 2016 study found that black Americans (the study did not address gender) are undertreated for pain compared to white Americans.[15] Here, in the UK, a 2016 study commissioned by Jo's Cervical Cancer Trust found that awareness of cervical cancer and how to prevent it is lower among women from a black and minority ethnic (BAME) background.[16] It's not too much of a leap to assume that today – like in the 1970s when Mantel was diagnosed with endometriosis – women of colour find it takes longer for their pain to be acknowledged, treated and diagnosed.

Vulvodynia is another chronic pain condition that torments women but is hugely misunderstood and under-researched. It involves a persistent pain in the vulva and is usually diagnosed after other conditions – recurring thrush yeast infections, Sjögren's syndrome (a disorder of the immune system that can cause vaginal dryness), STDs – have been eliminated. Essentially, vulvodynia is pain of the vulva when no clear cause can be identified.

The pain is usually stinging, tearing or tingling – and it

doesn't respond to painkillers like paracetamol or ibuprofen. It is sometimes, but not always, provoked by contact. It is estimated that as many as one in six women will suffer from vulvodynia at some point but it is a little-talked-about condition, presumably partly because we are still so bad at talking about vulvas.[17]

Women might feel too embarrassed to see a doctor – even when vulvodynia is getting in the way of sex (which can be excruciating) or even sitting (which can also be excruciating). If they do go to the doctor, they might encounter scepticism or bewilderment.

Rachael Revesz is a twenty-nine-year-old London-based journalist who regularly writes about living with vulvodynia. 'I want people to be able to read about another woman's experience with vulvodynia, to be able to find some information,' she says when I ask her why she is so keen to document it. When she first began experiencing vulval pain – 'a stabbing pain that's quite shallow, like a sharp instrument against the skin' – aged eighteen, she went to her local GP but quickly found herself facing a dead end. 'I started seeing doctors and I realized that wasn't going to help because they said things like I had a lack of hygiene, which was ridiculous.'

She eventually began to receive treatment – massage and exercises – that helped her manage the condition when someone recommended that she see a private physiotherapist who specialized in pelvic pain. 'Having it diagnosed has helped but it hasn't made it better,' Revesz says. 'They don't know what causes it. And they can't tell me when it's going to go away. My physio is very positive but I have to take her word for it.'

Revesz hopes that as more research into vulvodynia is conducted, there will be breakthroughs, but for now, she focuses on managing the condition rather than curing it. She regularly uses what she calls 'a wand', a curved glass instrument that she inserts into her vagina to 'stretch out the muscles and release pressure'. 'I have no idea if it works, maybe it's just a placebo,' she admits. And when she feels the aching that indicates a flare-up is imminent, she adjusts her lifestyle:

> I slow down and do as little as possible but it's difficult when your pelvis is connected to everything in your body – even if you turn around, even if you sit on the toilet, even if you cross your legs, even if you turn over in bed – everything you do will trigger it because everything is linked to your pelvis. So when you've got it really bad you've just got to not fear the pain.

Some women with vulvodynia or vestibulodynia (which is a similar condition but is confined to the vestibule) will find that antidepressants are the most effective form of treatment – drugs like the antidepressant amitriptyline can be used to treat vulval pain when administered at a lower dose. Local anaesthetic gel applied to the vulva can also help.

Sometimes vulvodynia and vestibulodynia are confused with vaginismus but, while there might be overlaps in symptoms, vaginismus is a separate condition. With vaginismus, the vagina tightens involuntarily when you try to insert something – a tampon, a finger, a penis, whatever – into it. Some people can use a tampon but not have penis-in-vagina sex; some people can have sex but it will be extremely painful; some people will find it impossible to insert anything at all. It's usually diagnosed after doctors rule out other possibilities, like an imperforate hymen.

Occasionally, people get vaginismus after they have previously had painless penetrative sex but usually it is a condition that people become aware of as a child or teenager. Shelby Hadden, who wrote and directed *Tightly Wound*, an animated short film about her experience of vaginismus, was fourteen when she sensed 'something was wrong'. 'When I was 14, I got my period – and I realized that I could not use a tampon,' she tells me. 'It felt like was no space in there, it was so painful, it just didn't feel right.'

Aged sixteen, she went to a doctor about her vaginismus and, over the next five years, she saw several specialists who offered her a variety of useless, sometimes creepy advice. 'I was told to drink alcohol when I wanted to be intimate with someone – and that was before I was even the legal age to do so,' she says. 'I had a doctor one time who refused to examine me because I wasn't sexually active.' (Hadden is from the US and was seeking treatment there, but her experience with getting a diagnosis and treatment for vaginismus is not unusual or particular to the US.)

Finding herself in a blind alley, she felt let down by doctors, as though they weren't listening to her, as though they doubted the veracity of her condition. 'It comes from a long history of dismissing women's pain,' she says, reflecting on the doctors' attitudes. 'It's easier to tell us that we're hysterical and it's all in our heads.'

She was twenty-one before she was referred to a physiotherapist and treatment commenced in earnest. Physiotherapy was a 'really lonely and frustrating experience at times' but after two years of exercises, of external and internal massage, of working with 'vaginal trainers' (tampon-shaped objects in varying sizes inserted into the vagina), she had penetrative sex for the first time.

Alongside the physiotherapy, Hadden had talking therapy – and that's often a key treatment for people with vaginismus. Psychosexual therapy can help those with vaginismus

understand their feelings about their body and sex, which might
be contributing to the condition. Vaginismus might be caused
by a bad sexual experience or by a fear that the vagina is too
small or a belief that sex is wrong or shameful.

Sometimes, though, therapy can simply offer support as
someone goes through physiotherapy, which can be a lonely
and isolating experience. 'It takes so long to see progress, or at
least it did for me, so it was really great to have someone to talk
through that with,' Hadden says. 'And I had a lot of anxieties
about sex and dating and dealing with an issue that people don't
know about or talk about.' She now considers herself 'for the
most part cured'.

Most women with vaginismus will seek treatment – and
some will see results within weeks of treatment beginning.
Other women will decide not to pursue or continue with treatment for vaginismus. They might decide that they can have a
fulfilling sex life without penetration, that they prefer to use
sanitary towels or period pants rather than tampons. Their vaginismus might cause problems if they need a cervical screening
test or if they want to become pregnant, but there are plenty of
people with vaginismus who live a happy and active life.

Rowan Ellis is a twenty-six-year-old queer woman, and first
realized she had vaginismus as a teenager. 'I've been extremely
lucky in that I do not need or want treatment for anything other
than medical reasons. I don't really mind not using tampons,'
she says. Having vaginismus doesn't have a negative effect on her
sex life:

I am queer and therefore have a different relationship
with penis-in-vagina sex than straight and cis people do.
The queerness for me makes it a non-issue because I don't
have the expectation that the main event in bed is going

to be one person putting this specific body part inside the other. I have found that in queer spaces there is often a lot more communication and freedom around what a fulfilling sex life looks like – and that penis-in-vagina sex doesn't have to be a part of it necessarily.

Ellis has never had a smear test but she will need to have one soon if she is to safeguard her own health. A general anaesthetic will be necessary, she suspects.

For the lucky among us, a smear test is a relatively straightforward procedure. It might be unpleasant, painful even, but we can take comfort in the fact that it's usually over quickly and has genuinely life-saving possibilities. Every year in the UK, smear tests prevent at least 2000 cervical cancer deaths. Cervical cancer is the most common cancer in women under thirty-five; in the UK, 3000 women a year are diagnosed with it and it kills about 850 women a year.[18]

Almost all cases of cervical cancer occur in women who have had the human papillomavirus (HPV), which is actually a group of viruses rather than a single type – there are more than 100 strains. Eighty per cent of people will contract HPV at some point in their lives[19] but it usually clears up on its own without any treatment; sometimes, though, the virus persists in the cervical cells and causes changes that can lead to them becoming cancerous.

There has, I think, been a reluctance to discuss HPV. We are so bad at talking about sex – and because sex and sexual contact is one of the ways in which the highly contagious HPV is spread, we have shied away from it. Smear tests have been almost mysterious; we have lain down half-naked on doctors' examination tables and felt an uncomfortable, strange pinch before waiting for letters that would tell us about changes or abnormal results or the need for repeated tests or colposcopies. We have not had the process explained clearly. A 2018 survey discovered that as many as 33 per cent of British women haven't even heard of HPV; 39 per cent of those surveyed would be worried what people thought of them if they were told they had HPV. A full 95 per cent of the women surveyed did not know that HPV could be contracted through protected sex, i.e. sex with a condom.[20]

The lack of clear information around HPV has left us without agency and contributed to a sense of unease, suspicion and even ambivalence about cervical screenings. Almost 40 per cent of women aged 25–29 chose not to attend a cervical screening test in 2017.[21] In 2018, it was revealed that screening rates were at their lowest for two decades.[22]

The HPV vaccine was introduced in England in 2008, with girls aged 12–13 routinely offered the vaccine for free with the NHS; it's been available to boys aged 12–13 since 2019. There have been individuals and groups, particularly in the US, that have opposed the widespread introduction of the vaccine, arguing that abstinence is better for protecting against HPV (the degree of anti-sex misogyny involved in that kind of thinking is off-the-charts levels of dangerous), but generally the vaccine has been an unmitigated success. It is vital, however, for all women, even those who were vaccinated as teenagers, to get cervical screening tests, as the vaccine does not protect against every strain of HPV.

From the late 2010s onwards, there have been changes to how cervical screening tests are carried out and pretty soon it will be the norm for primary HPV testing to occur. This means that all cervical screening samples will be tested for high-risk HPV first. (The screening will happen in the same way as before;

this change just affects what happens in the laboratory.) In cases where high-risk HPV is found, cytology (a study of the cells) will be carried out – if abnormal cells are seen, a colposcopy will be necessary.

If there are no abnormal cells, another cervical screening will be necessary in twelve months – most people will clear an HPV infection within a year.[23] This new system will reduce the number of repeat screenings a woman needs to have and research shows that a negative high-risk HPV result is a more reliable indicator that a woman will not develop cervical cancer than the previous method. It is estimated that, when fully implemented across England, HPV primary screening could prevent an additional 487 cases of cervical cancer a year.[24]

In cases where women do need a colposcopy, the doctor or specialist nurse will examine the cells of the cervix with a colposcope (like a microscope) and might take a biopsy. Abnormal cells can be removed during a colposcopy but sometimes a woman will need further treatment, with the abnormal cells being removed with laser treatment or a specialist excision process. If a woman is post-menopausal, has had all the children she wants or does not want children, doctors might recommend a hysterectomy, especially if the woman has had abnormal cells on her cervix more than once. If cervical cancer is diagnosed, radiotherapy or chemotherapy and surgery will likely be necessary.

Besides cervical cancer, there are four other types of gynaecological cancer. Womb cancer (sometimes called endometrial or uterine cancer) is the most common type of gynaecological cancer – over 9300 women are diagnosed with the disease in the UK each year. Ovarian cancer affects 7300 women in the UK each year. Women of any age can be diagnosed with ovarian and womb cancer but both are most common in post-menopausal women. Vulval and vaginal cancers are much rarer, affecting around 1000 and 250 women in the UK a year, respectively. Both are most common in women over sixty and the majority of cases of vulval and vaginal cancers are caused by HPV.[25] [26]

The symptoms of ovarian cancer include a feeling of fullness and persistent abdominal pain – symptoms will generally not be experienced in the vagina and vulva. With cervical, womb, vulval and vaginal cancers, symptoms may be experienced in the vagina and vulva. There might be strange bleeding, new pain, different discharge, unusual smells, sudden uncomfortable itching, lumps and swelling. If you have any of these symptoms, you must go to the doctor. And even if you feel like the doctor doesn't believe you, you must persist.

It could be uterine polyps or vulvodynia. It could be an STD like gonorrhoea or chlamydia. It could be thrush or BV. There are too many possibilities for me to name here; even as we set out to educate ourselves about our bodies, we know that we must leave so much to the experts, to the medics who are trained for this.

We must go and get tested. We must turn up for our cervical screenings. We must get to know our bodies, witness and observe the changes, report the inconsistencies and trust our instincts. If we come across a doctor who makes us feel stupid or scared, we should, if we can, request another. There are doctors and nurses and advocacy groups that will support us and help us and hear us.

The medical profession is changing; as recently as the 1980s, around 80 per cent of doctors were men. Now, more than half of all people who become doctors are women. (Those are UK figures; the stats are much more disappointing in some other countries.)[27] That's got to change something. It sounds basic but we have seen the seismic discoveries made by Australia's first female urologist, Helen O'Connell. Of course, people of any gender can be brilliant and compassionate doctors, talented and perceptive researchers, but I don't think it's reductive to assume that more work on the specifics of women's pain will occur when there are more female physicians and scientists.

Like I have said, *more research is needed* across so many areas involving women's health. In an environment where more people have vulvas and vaginas, where open and honest conversations about our vulvas and vaginas are taking place, that research is more likely to happen.

Through the bravery of women who show us their wounds, who speak about their pain, who tell us their stories, we can create the circumstances we need for change. When women can show their pain on their own terms – when they are showing the pain not just to be believed, but to demand more – women gain. When Hilary Mantel and Lena Dunham show us their pain, women gain. When Serena Williams writes about the haemorrhaging she experienced after childbirth; when Padma Lakshmi gives a speech about living with undiagnosed endometriosis; when the 'Call Your Girlfriend' podcast host Aminatou Sow talks frankly about being diagnosed with womb cancer, women gain. We gain knowledge and information and power. When pain isn't private, we are allowed to say, *That hurts*, we are allowed to demand that it doesn't hurt.

CHAPTER NINE

# Fertility, Teaching It
# and Talking About It

*Children are never simply themselves, co-extensive with
their own bodies, becoming alive to us when they turn in
the womb, or with their first unaided breath. Their lives
start long before birth, long before conception, and if
they are aborted or miscarried or simply fail to material-
ise at all, they become ghosts within our lives.*

Hilary Mantel, *Giving Up the Ghost: A Memoir*


My husband and I didn't have sex on our wedding night because we were exhausted, having spent a day drinking prosecco and making speeches and pledging everything we had to each other. We walked home from the wedding venue slowly, holding hands, and we fell asleep instantly, drunkenly; I was still wearing my dress. The next morning we put things right – we had sex, and afterwards, as we got dressed and had breakfast, I felt as though we had done something momentous. I was ovulating, according to my app, and I basked in the good timing. I had recently read a newspaper article about the power of hormones during the menstrual cycle and I thought, *How wonderful that I am ovulating during these twenty-four hours, how lucky I am to be experiencing higher levels of oestrogen right now, oestrogen that has made me sociable and relaxed and eloquent at my wedding.*

I thought, *How brilliant that I am ovulating and that I have just had sex with the man I love and that soon I will have a baby.*

It is humiliating to access that memory now, to look back on that blithe ignorance, that presumption of privilege.

A couple of days after our wedding, we went on honeymoon. We were in a small hotel on the island of Ischia when I got a terrible stomach bug. I was felled by it, by the vomiting and diarrhoea, crawling around the little hotel room that overlooked a dramatic bay. I writhed and hallucinated and my husband had to clean up after me, as I lay on the floor, spewing and sweating and seeing giant rabbits.

I thought, *The baby. This can't be good for the baby.*

But there was no baby.

I got my period shortly after we returned from honeymoon. I got my period every month for the next twelve months. And every month after that. I have my period as I write this sentence.

After the shock of the first period, I realized that I had only ever been taught about preventing pregnancy. I mean, yes, obviously, I had seen the ticking-biological-clock headlines but I was thirty-four when I got married. I had thought that I would squeeze in just before the thirty-five-and-your-fertility-is-done-for deadline. And anyway, I had read that the cliff we are all taught to fear isn't as steep as they make out. I had never been diagnosed with PCOS or endometriosis. I had fairly regular periods; sometimes they were a few days late but they always showed up. I had thought it was going to be easy.

In those first few months of not getting pregnant, I spent a lot of time on Internet forums, searching discussions for clues and hope. I would google things like 'negative pregnancy test but still no period' and I would find myself reading little messages written by women from New Zealand and America and Scotland. They offered hope to each other, or consolation, using platitudes and kindnesses and abbreviations.

A friend told me what 'TTC' meant. I had been saying 'unprotected sex with my husband'. She said that it's not called unprotected sex when you're aiming to get pregnant. 'It's called TTC,' she said, or 'trying to conceive'.

TTC sounded stupid but it was better than simply 'trying', a word with vast potential for joy or disappointment. It was less painful to say TTC, I found.


I learnt more than the lingo.

I learnt the facts of fertility. I already knew the basics – that a sperm fertilizes an egg, which is released from the ovaries. That it then travels along the fallopian tube to the womb, where it attaches itself to the endometrium. I knew that I ovulated once a month and that my vaginal discharge could offer me clues about my own fertility, that the stretchy clear discharge was the one that indicated I was at my most fertile time.

But I learnt more than the basics, more than I had been taught at school or picked up from magazines. From online forums and from books and from discussions with friends, I learnt and learnt.

I learnt about luteinizing hormone (LH) and how it indicates that you are about to ovulate. I learnt about the sticks that you can buy to test for LH, the way you can wee on them and wait for the two lines that indicate: go, go, go, have sex.

I learnt that an egg only lives for about twenty-four hours and that if it does not meet a sperm in that time, it disintegrates.

I learnt about the odds. About how, in one act of randomly timed sex, when both partners are healthy and no contraception is used, there is only a 3 per cent chance of conception. About how, when a woman aged about thirty-four or so is having regular, well-timed sex, there is a 20 per cent chance of conception each month.[1] I learnt about how those odds are affected by age – or I tried to, anyway, googling frantically, being served up wildly different information depending on which source I clicked on, which fear or hope I wanted confirmed.

I learnt that after a year of regular sex, around 84 per cent of couples will have become pregnant.[2] So after a year of the LH sticks and having sex when we didn't feel like it but thought that we should anyway, I learnt that we were unlucky. We were in the unlucky 16 per cent.

I learnt about resentment and disappointment. In pregnancy test adverts, the test is always positive. But all my tests were negative. And I felt stupid every time I did one, at work or on holiday or just before bed. I did them because my period was late but it never meant I was pregnant. And as I stood around waiting for the second blue line that I knew wasn't coming, I wished I hadn't bothered spending another £10 on this confirmation of disappointment.

I learnt that it felt lonely. Because even though I was lucky to be with someone I loved, he couldn't understand what I went through every month. He couldn't know what it felt like to analyse my own body, to scan it for twinges – was that pain the first sign of a period or was it an early indication of pregnancy, what the forums called 'implantation cramps'? He did not know what it felt like to look for the possibility of pregnancy in my breasts and my belly, inspecting their roundness and their fullness. He did not know the horror of PMS made worse by the disappointment of not being pregnant. He did not know what it meant to live in a body that might be pregnant or might not be pregnant, to feel that hope and terror every thirty days.

I learnt a new feeling that's close to jealousy, but feels different, at the same time. Every time a friend told me that she was pregnant, I was seized by it. 'It's just jealousy,' my husband would say, trying to comfort me. 'It's not jealousy,' I would scream and he would say sorry. I would wonder then, *Is it jealousy?* But it wasn't really jealousy; it was more like loneliness added upon loneliness. I had lost another one. She had happiness and hope and I felt like I couldn't keep telling her about my sadnesses now.

I learnt that it gets less shocking, less upsetting, month by month by month. It is still sad but I learnt that I am stronger than I thought I was.

All of this learning begs the question: shouldn't we be teaching this stuff? Shouldn't we include more information about fertility, much more, in our sex education? And it's not just me asking. The notion of including information about fertility in RSE has been floated by several experts in recent years. Each time an individual or an organization campaigns for fertility to be included in school curriculums – pointing out the pain of involuntary childlessness, the falling fertility rates, the misinformation that surrounds in vitro fertilization (IVF) and egg freezing – the headlines are similar.

'"Girls as young as NINE should be taught about fertility": Experts say children should be warned of starting a family too late' – that's from the *Daily Mail*.[3] 'Teach girls how to get pregnant, say doctors' – that's from *The Times*.[4]

And each time I see those headlines, I wince. Firstly, why just *girls*? The experts always say that we should teach *children* about fertility but the newspapers always say *girls*. And secondly, I wonder, well, would it even help? If women are putting off pregnancy (and statistics show that they are), hasn't that got more to do with the economic reality of life after the 2008 financial crash than a lack of information about how ageing affects our fertility?

Four years before I started trying to have a baby, I experienced an unplanned pregnancy. I was with the same partner but our circumstances were different. And it wasn't just that we weren't married yet or that we hadn't been on an Italian honeymoon. It wasn't just that we hadn't got all our ducks in a row. Our ducks were all over the place. We didn't live together; we lived with flatmates in shared accommodation. We had only been together a few months. We had no money. The website I was working at had just been shut down and I had lost my job. We didn't know what to do. We had an abortion.

I made the decision to have an abortion even though I knew that, in different, better circumstances, I wanted a baby. I wanted a baby even then, in those bad circumstances, but it didn't feel possible.

So the thought of teaching nine-year-olds about their fertility seems troubling to me. I was aware of the basics of fertility when I was thirty-one but I had an abortion because I could not afford to continue with the pregnancy. How do we teach nine-year-olds about *that*?

In the years that followed the unplanned pregnancy and abortion, I set about lining up my ducks. I worked hard to earn more money. I moved in with my boyfriend and we worked on making our relationship strong and durable. We got married in front of friends and family in a deconsecrated church a mile or so from our flat. It was the sunniest August bank holiday since the 1980s that day's papers announced.

But when our ducks were in a row, we tried to have a baby and it didn't happen.

Would I have made a different decision about whether to have an abortion at thirty-one if I had had fertility classes at school? Probably not. Would I have made a different decision if I had been more supported – financially and holistically – by the state and employers? Almost certainly.

To fully examine the notion of whether fertility should be taught at schools, I must look beyond myself. According to the experts, there are people who are uncertain about fertility and how it declines with age; there are people who see celebrities becoming mothers at fifty-five and think, *That could be me.*

Professor Geeta Nargund is the founder and medical director of CREATE Fertility, a private fertility clinic, and is a senior consultant gynaecologist and lead consultant for reproductive medicine services at St George's Hospital, London. She passionately believes that we should teach young people about fertility and regularly visits schools to talk to teenagers about how their fertility is affected by age, diet, STDs and other factors.

As a doctor specializing in reproductive medicine, she is accustomed to seeing the grief that accompanies infertility. She wants as few people as possible to experience that grief. She wants all teenagers to be taught about preventing pregnancy *and* planning pregnancy. 'What we want to do is make sure we can give that nuanced message about both sides of the coin,' she tells me. 'On the one side, protecting your fertility; on the other side, preventing pregnancy. They are both sides of the same coin, you know, contraception and conception, and that nuanced message needs to be understood.'

Professor Nargund doesn't say that her ambition to educate teenagers about fertility is the only way to address the falling fertility rates; she acknowledges that economic and social factors play a huge part. But she believes that sex education must be updated to reflect the fact that one in seven couples struggles to conceive.[5]

She says:

> I see women and couples every day of my life, and many, many women don't know how fast [fertility] can decline. When you look at the detail, when you look at the reality, there are gaps in knowledge. When you fill them, that helps. Education is never about pressure or anxiety, education is to relieve anxiety. That is the bottom line. I don't think anybody could convince me or argue with me about 'if you educate, you're going to create anxiety'. In fact what is desperately needed is to educate and give girls and women that very balanced, up-to-date, evidence-based scientific information in a language they understand.

Jessica Hepburn is another woman who believes that fertility should be taught at schools. Hepburn is not a medical expert – she is a writer and theatre producer – but after eleven rounds of unsuccessful IVF, she thinks she can offer an important insight into infertility and its consequences. Hepburn began to try for a baby when she was in her mid-thirties (she is now in her late forties) and she wants to tell teenagers that, in her particular set of circumstances, that did not leave her enough time. She wants to teach young people that fertility declines with age, that it is harder for a woman to get pregnant in her thirties than it is in her twenties or teens.

She says:

Ninety-nine per cent of young women would say that they want a family – but not now. If they're getting better education now, at least they'll be more prepared for the challenges they might face. I'm driven by that. I have information that I didn't know at their age and I would be doing the next generation a disservice if I didn't tell them. They can do what they want with that information.

Hepburn also thinks that egg freezing – the process of retrieving a woman's eggs and preserving them for use at a later time – should be offered to young women. 'I think young people should have egg freezing loans in the way that they have student loans,' she says. When women freeze eggs later in their lives – in their late thirties, say – the eggs are not as likely to result in a successful pregnancy.[6]

As well as educating young people, Hepburn wants to promote a more honest conversation about fertility. At a time when more single women are pursuing motherhood with the help of donor sperm, when LGBTQ+ families are opening up about their experiences and routes to parenthood, when there are more options than ever before, many people still find it difficult to talk about infertility and fertility treatments.

There are several taboos that lead to silence or squeamishness. Most obviously, there is the issue of sex, of vaginas, of wombs, of women's bodies. We are not good at talking about sex and vaginas and wombs and women's bodies – and, by extension, fertility – with any degree of impartiality or honesty. Then there is the issue of failure, says Hepburn. It is difficult to discuss our failures, our natural inclination is to hide them away, and infertility can feel like a failure.

Another taboo, Hepburn suggests, is to do with feminism:

We are the generation who thought we could have it all. My generation – and women a little bit older and younger than me – we had the pill, we had legalized abortion, we went to university, we got on the career ladder. We left it late, sometimes too late, to start a family. And I think it's really hard to say that.

For me, that stings, that idea that I might have left it 'too late', and I feel myself bristle: haven't men left it too late, too?

Professor Nargund is adamant that boys and girls must be taught about fertility at the same time: 'From the beginning, it [must be] both boys and girls – both of them are important when it comes to making a baby.' But, she admits, there is a lot less chatter about men's 'biological clocks' than there is about women's. 'Both men and women are equally responsible and contribute equally when it comes to reproduction and making babies, but because the "biological clock" ticks faster for women, I suppose society talks about it. But when it comes to taking responsibility for your own fertility, it is for both men and women, which is why we need to educate both.'

Perhaps, it is even more urgent that we educate boys and men about fertility. They are not the ones with vaginas and wombs and so they have not faced a barrage of media reports about their 'ticking biological clocks'. But fertility declines in men as well as women – and there is striking evidence to suggest that men's fertility is declining overall, with environmental factors being blamed. A study published by the Hebrew University of Jerusalem in 2017 suggested that sperm count among Western men had more than halved over the previous forty years.[7] Hagai Levine, an epidemiologist and lead author of the study, said at the time: 'The results are quite shocking... This is a classic under-the-radar huge public health problem that is really neglected.'

What is even more taboo than vaginas and wombs and sex? Men's infertility, it seems. Even the way in which we describe conception is framed around some super-masculine sperm racing and competing to fertilize a docile egg. As pointed out by the anthropologist Emily Martin in her 1991 academic article, 'The Egg and the Sperm: How Science Has Constructed a Romance Based on Stereotypical Male-Female Roles', the egg is actually much more aggressive than it's traditionally been described and has a competition of its own in the ovary before it's released.[8]

When we talk about infertility, it is so often in relation to women and their ovaries. And that makes sense: infertility in women is commonly caused by problems with ovulation, resulting from PCOS or thyroid problems or premature ovarian failure or endometriosis. But in as many as half of all couples experiencing non-age-related infertility, abnormal semen quality or male sexual dysfunction is the cause.[9] So, around half the time, it's not about the ovaries, it's about the sperm – and that's an issue that's getting worse not better as sperm count falls around the world. It's an issue that should be splashed on front pages and discussed on radio phone-in shows, but it's an issue that is not widely discussed – because the notion of men's virility is too powerful to question.

There isn't enough research being carried out into the causes of falling sperm count – and into cures for male infertility – because men's infertility is unmentionable. There isn't enough support being offered to men experiencing infertility because men's infertility is unmentionable.

152

It is relatively easy to cover up, too. When a miscarriage occurs because of abnormal sperm, it happens in the woman's body. When IVF is required because of abnormal sperm, it happens in the woman's body. I do not point this out to make men feel bad about their infertility. I point this out to say that ideas and myths of male virility harm men *and* women, and should be challenged.

There is a 2013 article from *The Atlantic* magazine that my friends and I have shared with each other over the years. It is titled 'How Long Can You Wait to Have a Baby?' and over several thousand words, its author, Jean M. Twenge, sets out to investigate whether women's fertility really does dramatically decline at thirty-five like we've been told it does.[10]

Twenge points out that so much of the information we are given about infertility is unreliable. 'The widely cited statistic that one in three women ages 35 to 39 will not be pregnant after a year of trying,' Twenge writes, 'is based on an article published in 2004 in the journal *Human Reproduction*. Rarely mentioned is the source of the data: French birth records from 1670 to 1830.'

She draws attention to the fact that many fertility experts see patients who are experiencing fertility problems – and while success rates for IVF might be significantly higher for younger patients, the same might not be true for natural conception. 'Studies of natural conception are surprisingly difficult to conduct – that's one reason both IVF statistics and historical records play an outsize role in fertility reporting,' writes Twenge, who became a mother three times after turning thirty-five.

It is a great article: interesting, thorough, well-researched. It is a rebuff to the media reports about selfish career women who 'left it too late'. That's why my friends and I sent it to each other: we were comforted by it, buoyed by it – as we broke up with unsuitable partners, as we saved up for deposits on houses, as we fought for better pay, as we 'put off' motherhood.

I am thirty-five now. When I arrange a dinner, I check to see whether there are high chairs and baby-changing facilities at the restaurant. It happened suddenly but now lots of my friends have babies. There are friends who got pregnant the first time they tried, and they tell me, blushing, embarrassed by their good fortune. There are friends for whom it took months and months, and they wondered if it would ever happen and then it did. There are friends who had miscarriages. There are friends who have had IVF. And there are friends who have used donor eggs and donor sperm.

At the dinners, there are some of us who will never have babies – because of biology or circumstances or love or luck or choice. And I wonder: what could we be taught? Would a fertility education change any of this?

After a year of TTC, my husband and I were sent for tests.

My blood tests showed that I ovulated – everything seemed to be working fine. Scans and a hysteroscopy showed that I had some fibroids and a tilted womb but it was nothing that was likely to be affecting my fertility, according to the doctors.

My husband's test results showed abnormalities. There was no sperm in his semen – it's a condition called azoospermia and it affects around one in 100 men. We knew that he had had sperm in his semen before. We had got pregnant before. But, it seems that illness (he had contracted tuberculosis in the months after we got married) had affected his urogenital system and his fertility.

Our story doesn't have a neat ending. It's ongoing. It involves urologists and gynaecologists. It might involve a type of IVF procedure called intracytoplasmic sperm injection (ICSI). It might involve donor sperm or adoption. We don't know yet. We are figuring it out.

The diagnosis of azoospermia means that I have stopped cursing myself, I have stopped admonishing myself, I have stopped tormenting myself about having left it *too late*. Every month, I continue to feel a sharp disappointment as my period arrives, even though it's now expected – but having a diagnosis, and one that feels shared between my husband and me, makes it easier. It's better than not knowing. It's better than feeling that I was wrong, selfish, overly confident to have left it *too late*.

Lots of people facing infertility never get a diagnosis: some people have IVF not knowing why they couldn't conceive naturally. IVF doesn't work for some people, even after eleven rounds, with the fertility doctors adjusting the treatment as they go.

So even if we decide to teach children and teenagers about fertility, there will be unknowns. Those of us who have experienced infertility attempt to become experts, sitting in the glow of our laptops searching for answers and clues and case studies online, but even the experts, the actual experts, are baffled a lot of the time. So what could we tell children and teenagers with certainty? What *do* we know?

We know about ovarian reserve, how girls are born with all the eggs they will ever have, hundreds and hundreds of thousands of them – and how they begin losing them while still in utero.

We know that women's fertility decreases with age – but we know that it varies greatly from woman to woman. We know, with certainty, that it is harder for women to get pregnant in their forties than in their twenties – but we also know that some women will have successful pregnancies in their forties and some women will face infertility in their twenties.

We actually *know* that fertility doesn't *fall off a cliff* at thirty-five but we pretend that we don't know that.

We know that the IVF success rates are higher for younger women.

We know that sperm count is falling – but we don't know why.

We know that we don't know enough about infertility, female or male.

We know that infertility is painful, that it can negatively impact mental health, that it can damage relationships.

We know that infertility is expensive, ruinously so for some.

We know that not everyone who wants a biological baby will be able to have one.

Can that be taught? Well, we could give it a try.

At the moment, it feels like the conversation about fertility focuses on a woman's body – but we need to talk about more than that. Let's talk about the mental health implications of infertility and how we can support people experiencing that. Let's talk about the unethical businesses that spring up around infertility and how we can regulate the industry more effectively. Let's talk about the cost of childcare and the housing crisis and how those factors force people to delay parenthood. Let's talk about race and religion and how infertility is particularly taboo in some cultures. Let's talk about how some people simply don't want to have kids.

Jean M. Twenge's advice that women hoping to get pregnant in their thirties shouldn't panic is good advice. Professor Geeta Nargund's advice that teenagers be taught more about the science of fertility is good advice. We are made to feel like those pieces of advice contradict each other but they don't have to.

Because at the heart of any conversation about fertility, there must surely be an acknowledgement that it's complicated.

We were all taught the story of the sperm meeting an egg but a fertility re-education must be broader and thornier. A fertility re-education must examine the ambitions of women; it must interrogate the ways in which we seek to control women's sexuality; it must, if it is going to work at all, be frank about the realities of women's lives. A discussion of men's fertility must be included in any fertility re-education.

And even then, even if we succeed in creating a discourse around fertility that is honest and expansive and allows for contradictions and complications, we must accept that there will be lessons that will be impossible to teach. There are lessons my younger self could never have learnt. With fertility, there are lessons in which there are no right answers, no wrong questions.

CHAPTER TEN

# Getting Pregnant,
# and What Comes Next

*I'm a means, a stage, a cow in calf.*
*I've eaten a bag of green apples,*
*Boarded the train there's no getting off.*

Sylvia Plath, 'Metaphors'

Weight gain; sore breasts; bleeding throughout the
month; irritability; depression; a decreased sex drive; an
increased likelihood of developing potentially fatal blood clots;
a link to breast cancer.

The possible side effects of hormonal contraception – such
as the pill, the implant, the vaginal ring or the hormonal IUS –
can be off-putting, frightening even. Despite that, millions and
millions of us have, for decades, relied on it. (The contraceptive
pill was first introduced in the US in 1960 and it became available in the UK the following year.)[1] In countries where hormonal
contraception is available and affordable, it has probably been
the single most significant development in the lives of the women
who live there, allowing us to have heterosexual penetrative sex

without worrying about the possibility of an unplanned pregnancy. (Although it is important to note that no contraception is 100 per cent effective.)

There are benefits to hormonal contraception that go beyond not getting pregnant, too: it can halt periods (and period pain and PMS); it can help clear acne; it can be used to treat endometriosis and PCOS; it can help prevent against bowel, ovarian and womb cancer.[2]

Weighing up the pros and cons of hormonal contraception can be difficult, however, and although 'mood swings' doesn't look like much written down, it can feel debilitating when experienced by the individual. Crying almost every day or feeling sudden and unexplained anger can disrupt women's whole lives, even if 'mood swings' just appears in a tiny font in a long list on a lightweight piece of paper that comes wedged in the box of contraceptive pills.

Currently, there are only two types of male contraception. Condoms have the benefit of being highly effective at protecting against HIV and most STDs (although not ones spread by skin-to-skin contact) but are often not favoured by couples in long-term relationships. And a vasectomy – a surgical procedure that prevents sperm from reaching semen – is only suitable for men who have decided that they will not want children in the future.

At the time of writing, almost sixty years after the widespread introduction of female hormonal contraception, there is nowhere in the world where male hormonal contraception is available. There are drugs in development but some trials have been halted due to side effects experienced by the men taking part. Side effects include acne, mood disorders and changes in libido – complaints that many point out are regularly experienced by women who use hormonal contraception.[3]

Increasingly, women frustrated by hormonal contraception are turning to 'natural contraception'. In 2018 the US Food & Drug Administration (FDA) approved the use of the Natural Cycles app as a contraceptive. This approval of the first digital contraceptive was seen as historic – and controversial. The app – which, at the time of writing, costs £40 a year – tracks a woman's menstrual cycle and daily temperature (which you measure and log yourself) and then uses an algorithm to identify the most and least fertile times. It can be used for birth control or for planning a family and it is, essentially, a modern updating of the fertility-awareness methods that have been around for a century, including the Catholic Church-recommended rhythm method. The woman behind the app, Elina Berglund, is a young Swedish physicist, with top-notch scientific credentials and a knack for public relations. She promotes her product via TED Talks and press interviews; there are ads for Natural Cycles on Facebook and Instagram.

In December 2017, it was reported that more than 125,000 British women were using the app and that, consequently, sales of the contraceptive pill had dropped.[4] The marketing had worked. But soon there were questions about whether the app itself worked. In January 2018, the app was reported to the Swedish authorities after a single hospital saw thirty-seven women who needed abortions after relying on Natural Cycles for contraception.[5]

In July 2018, the British novelist Olivia Sudjic wrote a newspaper article about getting pregnant and having an abortion while using the digital contraceptive.[6] In August 2018, the same month the FDA approved it, the UK's Advertising Standards Authority (ASA) banned a Natural Cycles advert, contending that claims that it was 'highly accurate' and 'provided a clinically tested alternative to other birth control methods' were misleading.[7]

Natural Cycles responded to the controversies by pointing out that it has been cleared by the FDA and claiming that the app is 93 per cent effective with typical use.

I was one of 120,000 women in Britain who began using Natural Cycles during 2017. I knew that I was planning to start a family soon so I bought the app to try to get to know my own body, uncontrolled by the pill, a little more. Among those of us who spent most of our teens and early adulthood on hormonal contraception, there is a sense that we don't know our bodies, our cycles; we don't know what's normal for us; we don't know how hormones affect our sex drives, our moods, our appearance, our fertility. And this app – sleek and 'natural' and easy to use – offered an education. The lack of side effects was also an obvious boon.

What perhaps hasn't been made explicit enough in the advertising of Natural Cycles is how the reliability of 'natural contraception' is affected by factors like hangovers (alcohol affects body temperature) and PCOS (irregular ovulation is difficult to track). And I know that if I had a friend for whom an unplanned pregnancy would spell disaster, I would prefer to think she was on the pill rather than trusting an app.

Hormonal contraception is not going anywhere – estimates suggest that the industry behind the contraceptive pill will be worth \$23 billion by 2023.[8] But the industry should note how eager hundreds of thousands of women were to abandon the pill as soon as a digital alternative arrived. Women have doubts, women have questions, women are seeking an alternative.

When contraception isn't used during sex or when contraception fails, pregnancy can occur. That is a fact that underpins our lives. Even as birth rates fall in the UK, Europe and the US, more than 80 per cent of women in England and Wales will become mothers, according to data collected in 2016.[9]

It's hard to track down the exact figures but we must assume that even more women will actually get pregnant but not become mothers, due to abortion and miscarriage.

Globally, one in four pregnancies ends in abortion – half of those are thought to be illegal.[10] Tens of thousands of women die each year after having an abortion in countries where it is illegal.[11] Abortion has been legal up to twenty-four weeks gestation in the UK (except for Northern Ireland) since 1967 and one in three women in the UK will have an abortion in her lifetime. The vast majority – a full 92 per cent – of the abortions carried out in the UK occur before thirteen weeks gestation. More than 80 per cent take place before ten weeks gestation. Medical abortions – which can take place in the first ten weeks of pregnancy and involve taking pills that induce a miscarriage – are increasingly common, accounting for 62 per cent of all abortions in the UK in 2016.[12]

Since 2018, women in England, Scotland and Wales have been allowed to take the second pill in a medical abortion at home so that the worst symptoms – heavy bleeding and painful cramps – can happen in a place where they feel comfortable.

There are two types of surgical abortions. With a vacuum or suction aspiration, which is used up to fifteen weeks of gestation, a tube is inserted through the cervix and into the womb and suction is used to remove the pregnancy. It usually takes five to ten minutes. With a dilatation and evacuation (D&E), the cervix is dilated and forceps are used to remove the pregnancy. It usually takes about ten to twenty minutes. Late-term abortions are extremely rare – less than 1 per cent of abortions occur after twenty-two weeks gestation and generally they are carried out when there is a considerable chance that a foetus will not survive outside the womb or that a child will be born with 'significant handicaps'.[13]

Ninety-five per cent of women who have an abortion do not regret it.[14] Plenty of women will find the experience upsetting and even heartbreaking – I know that I did – but very few women will regret having an abortion. I had an abortion and I went on to experience the pain of infertility and, while sometimes that feels like a strange dichotomy, I don't regret having an abortion. Regret is not a tool that allows us to rearrange history and tinker with our timelines and change our circumstances – and I think that most women who have an abortion understand that.

When a woman has an abortion for a medical reason – because of a fatal foetal abnormality that means the baby will not survive outside the womb, for example – she might feel that it is more fitting to speak about it as pregnancy or baby loss. So, too, might women who have ectopic pregnancies: one in eighty to ninety pregnancies are ectopic pregnancies[15] (where the fertilized egg implants outside the womb) and these pregnancies will have to be ended with surgery or medication.

It is estimated that as many as one in four pregnancies end in miscarriage – some will occur before a woman even knows that she is pregnant. A miscarriage that occurs before a gestational sac is visible on an ultrasound, but after a blood test or at-home pregnancy test has confirmed a pregnancy, is called a chemical pregnancy. Among women who know they are pregnant, the miscarriage figure is one in six. The majority of miscarriages will happen in the first trimester, and a miscarriage that occurs before thirteen weeks gestation is called an 'early miscarriage'. A 'late miscarriage' is rare and happens from weeks fourteen to twenty-four of pregnancy. A miscarriage after twenty-four weeks is a stillbirth.[16] Symptoms of a miscarriage might include heavy vaginal bleeding, unusual discharge, pain or a loss of pregnancy symptoms. Sometimes there are no signs that a miscarriage has occurred and a woman will only find out after having a routine scan. This is called a 'missed miscarriage' or a 'silent miscarriage'. Miscarriages must often be managed – sometimes women will wait and allow the miscarriage to occur naturally, but this can take weeks, and some women prefer to arrange for a medical or surgical procedure.

There are various factors that can lead to a miscarriage but the majority of early miscarriages are due to chromosomal abnormalities in the foetus.[17] The chances of chromosomal abnormalities increase with maternal age; so too does the chance of miscarriage. Studies have shown that many people underestimate the frequency of miscarriage while misunderstanding the causes, with women blaming themselves or their lifestyle choices. They might worry that stress, exercise, drinking a glass of wine or eating the wrong thing played a part; a 2015 survey revealed that 21 per cent of people mistakenly thought that getting into an argument could cause a woman to have a miscarriage.[18] But in the vast majority of miscarriages, nothing could have been done differently.

Repeated miscarriages are uncommon but 1 per cent of women experience recurrent miscarriage, which is generally defined as the loss of three or more consecutive pregnancies. Causes for recurrent miscarriage include infection and thrombophilic (blood-clotting) defects, uterine problems and cervical 'weakness', but often doctors can find no reason. Late miscarriage can be caused by chromosomal abnormalities, by infection, by anatomical problems like cervical 'weakness' or an unusually shaped womb.

Although miscarriage is the most common complication in pregnancy, affecting as many as one in four women, it has, traditionally, not been something we speak about regularly or openly in Europe and the US. There is a custom that pregnancy is not announced until twelve weeks gestation, after the first scan, and what happens before that is private: the debilitating nausea, the constipation and the fatigue, the fretting, the hope and excitement. Some pregnant women prefer it that way: they might be superstitious or they might fear that if they do go on to experience miscarriage, they could not face the querying and sympathetic faces. As most miscarriages are early miscarriages they happen in this time of *unannounced* pregnancy. The miscarriages themselves are *unannounced*, too – private, lonely, often taboo.

For many women, miscarriage is one of the most painful and upsetting experiences they will face in life: ensuing depression and post-traumatic stress disorder are common.[19]

The lack of frank and open conversation does not help. Myths about the causes of miscarriage are more likely to propagate without frank and open conversation. Funding for research into miscarriage, and how to prevent it, is less likely to be raised without frank and open conversation. We must ask ourselves why we expect women to remain quiet about this loss, why we keep the discussion around miscarriage so muted. The squeamishness around women's bodies surely contributes to the quietness. The misogynistic sense that women are meant for motherhood plays a part, too: in pregnancy, the woman is woman and child; after miscarriage, she is *just woman* again. And her story, her womanly story of pain and loss and blood, is ignored.

When writing about experiencing miscarriage, Maggie O'Farrell explored the idea of grief after pregnancy loss. She wrote her womanly story, pain and loss and blood and all. She asked why women should be expected to stay silent – and she concluded that they shouldn't:

There is a school of thought out there that expects women to get over a miscarriage as if nothing has happened, to metabolize it quickly and get on with life. It's just like a bad period, a friend of mine was told, briskly, by her mother-in-law.

To this, I say: Why? Why should we carry on as if it's nothing out of the ordinary? It is not ordinary to conceive a life and then to lose it; it's very far from ordinary.[20]

Miscarriage is common – but it is not ordinary.

Despite abortion and miscarriage being common, more common than perhaps we are comfortable acknowledging, in the majority of pregnancies, a woman will go on to have a baby.

Almost immediately, she will notice changes in her body – her breasts will swell; she will have headaches; she might notice a metallic taste in her mouth; morning sickness will descend making car journeys and hot rooms torture; she will develop food cravings and aversions; she will suddenly be unable to stomach apples or cheese or fish or whatever. She will be constipated, faint, exhausted. She will get nosebleeds. Changes happen in the vagina too: she will notice more discharge, which her vagina creates for increased protection against bacteria. Later, as the pregnancy progresses, her vulva will become heavy and full, uncomfortably so, perhaps. She will have varicose veins in the vulva, especially if this isn't her first pregnancy. Towards the end of pregnancy, she will see pink-streaked mucus in her pants: this is the mucus that has been plugging the cervix – sometimes called 'the show' and indicates that birth is imminent.

All of these symptoms and signs and stages will differ from woman to woman. Not everyone will experience everything on

that list. Some women will escape morning sickness and varicose veins and nosebleeds; others won't notice too much change
in their discharge or their appetites. Pregnancy obviously has
some undeniable biological realities that apply to every single
pregnant person, but pregnancy differs from person to person,
and from first pregnancy to second or third.

I grew up thinking that fertility, pregnancy and childbirth
were standardized, one-size-fits-all states. Conception occurred
as soon as a straight couple had sex without using contraception; pregnancy was plotted over nine months with regular and
predictable markers along the way; childbirth was the same
for everyone – and whether you had an epidural or a caesarean
depended on your personal preferences rather than the circumstances of the birth.

It is only recently that I have realized how unique each person's situation is, how wrong I was in my assumptions. Around
three years ago, my friends started to have babies and when I
went round to their houses and cradled these little infants they
had created, they told me about childbirth.

Sometimes it had taken a couple of hours, sometimes a couple of days; some friends described it as no big deal, 'like really
bad period pain'; some of them had been in serious medical
danger. I was already (I think, I hope) suspicious of the value
judgements applied to how women give birth (with an epidural
or by caesarean section or 'naturally'), but, listening to my
friends as they fed dozing newborns, made me realize how truly
odious so much of the conversation about childbirth is.

It dawned on me that until my own close friends started having babies, I'd never really heard any birth stories. We don't talk
about pregnancy and birth, certainly not the nitty-gritty of it.

Rebecca Schiller, the author of two books about pregnancy
and the founder of Birthrights, a charity that promotes human

rights in pregnancy and childbirth, agrees that we just hear one story, stripped of all complications:

> No one wants to talk about vaginas, really. So the only way we can talk about it is to make it simple and uniform – you know, 'This is what will happen to you.' The idea that everybody might have completely, wildly different experiences is just too much for the world at the moment.

So our squeamishness about women's bodies means that we flatten out and package up the weeks and months of pregnancy, the hours and days of childbirth. We attempt to make them standard because we don't *listen* to women about pregnancy and childbirth; we *tell* them about pregnancy and childbirth.

It is a disempowering strategy, one that robs women of autonomy and confidence. A new, more honest strategy would empower women.

Schiller says:

> Some people will find it challenging, but actually having a mixture of good support and good information throughout pregnancy, birth and afterwards, is the key. It's helpful for women to understand what their rights are, to understand that there are things they can ask for, that their wishes should be respected, and that's based in the law. That can be powerful for them.

When people are making birth plans – a record for the maternity team about preferences during labour and birth – they should bear in mind their personal circumstances. Women who have had vaginismus or vulvodynia or who have experienced sexual abuse or violence might have specific needs in pregnancy and childbirth. Women who are disabled or who have had a prior traumatic experience during pregnancy and childbirth will have particular requirements, too. Trans and non-binary people might find it useful to create a detailed birth plan, outlining their circumstances and wishes. If someone is planning a birth that isn't standard, it is useful to get the plan agreed with midwives and doctors in advance. Of course, though, birth doesn't always go to plan.

Being aware of the various ways that childbirth can occur, of the multiple paths there are to delivering a healthy baby, can feel overwhelming for some women; there might be a sense that they do not want to hear rare 'horror stories' and would rather focus on the positive. This is understandable, but some women argue that hearing and recognizing a range of birth stories will help them feel prepared and in control.

A friend, who has one young child and is pregnant with her second, puts it this way:

> People should be encouraged to picture and anticipate all of the most common birth experiences, beyond the one they want for themselves. Birth plans are all well and good, but once you get attached to one way of doing things, it can close you off to looking into what happens if things don't go according to plan – which is likely. There is a line of thinking that you shouldn't listen to 'negative' birth stories as that will make it harder for you to have a 'positive' birth. I think this is bullshit – the more informed you are, the more power you have and the less surprised you will be.

Cradling all those newborns, I looked at their tiny noses, their dinky feet and ears. They felt almost weightless in my arms.

They were so, so little. And yet the realization that a baby, small as she may be, passes through the vagina will probably always feel sort of preposterous to someone who has not yet experienced childbirth. It just doesn't feel possible that the vaginal opening could accommodate a baby's head. But it is: the perineum – the area of skin and muscle between the vagina and the anus – stretches to accommodate the baby. Often, it will tear; in fact, most women will tear to some extent. If the skin tears, it might heal without stitches, but if skin and muscle is torn, stitches will probably be necessary. Women are encouraged to massage the perineum, externally and via the vagina, towards the end of pregnancy in preparation for birth. Using a perineal warm compress during the pushing stage of labour can also help minimize tears.

Sometimes an episiotomy – which is a cut in the perineum to widen the opening – is necessary. Today, up to 19 per cent of women in the UK have an episiotomy during childbirth, with the number being significantly higher for first-time mothers.[21] An episiotomy might be necessary if the baby appears to be in distress; if there is a clinical need for the use of forceps or a ventouse suction cup; if the baby is very large; if it is a breech birth, with the baby being born legs first; if the mother is exhausted; or if a speedy birth is necessary to keep her and the baby safe. Compared to a tear, an episiotomy will generally involve more blood loss, be more painful and take longer to heal. A woman should always be asked to consent to an episiotomy but unfortunately that doesn't always happen, in hospitals in the UK and around the world.

The episiotomy has a controversial history: introduced in the eighteenth century, it didn't become a common practice until the 1930s when an American doctor, Joseph DeLee, sometimes nauseatingly called the 'father of modern obstetrics', advocated for its widespread introduction. By 1979, episiotomies were performed in 63 per cent of vaginal births in the US.[22] In the UK, the figure was around 50 per cent in 1979.[23] Doctors tended to write off episiotomies as a 'little snip', underestimating the seriousness of the procedure and the implications it had on women's health, but the practice had its critics.

One of the most prominent opponents to routine episiotomy was Sheila Kitzinger, who railed against the medicalization of childbirth. Kitzinger was highly influential – when she died aged eighty-six in 2015, the *Guardian* obituary noted that: 'She could reasonably be said to have done more than anyone else to change attitudes to childbirth in the past 50 years'[24] – and she is perhaps best known in the UK as the founder of the National Childbirth Trust (NCT). Writing in 1979, Kitzinger observed that: 'The evidence for the routine or liberal use of episiotomy is unconvincing. Episiotomy is an example of an intervention which has been introduced into obstetric practice without accurate assessment and without asking women what they prefer.'[25]

During the course of her career as the author of more than thirty books on pregnancy and childbirth, Kitzinger argued that birth could be an ecstatic, even orgasmic, experience. It was a stance that raised eyebrows and, while she always used language that was non-judgemental, some women felt that Kitzinger was opposed to epidurals (an anaesthetic injected into the spine) or elective caesarean sections.

This conflict was played up in the media and there is sometimes a sense that there are two camps in childbirth: the 'just put yourself out of your misery and get the epidural' crowd versus the 'I'm going to float through childbirth anaesthetized by my own orgasms' gang. But it's a whole lot more complicated than that. There is a link between having an epidural and the need for an episiotomy because an epidural is likely to prolong labour – but often women who were sure that they would not opt for an epidural or episiotomy find that they do, when the time comes. Their labour goes on for days or their baby appears to be distressed. And they do whatever is right and best for them. The most important thing is that women should be consulted about episiotomies, their consent should be asked and they should receive adequate aftercare.

There is no *easy* way to give birth, although people like to pretend that there is. The phrase 'too posh to push' is sometimes bandied about when women have caesarean sections, which account for over 20 per cent of births in the UK – perhaps because C-sections are more expensive for the hospital than a vaginal birth; perhaps because Victoria 'Posh Spice' Beckham delivered her four children via C-section; perhaps because older mothers, who are likely to be wealthier than younger mothers, are more likely to need a C-section.[26] Whatever the origin of the phrase, it is obscene to suggest that the delivery of a baby via a major operation – an operation that saves the lives of mothers and babies every single day – is some sort of luxury.

A caesarean is either elective (planned) or emergency (only decided once labour is underway) and involves a cut, just below the bikini line, through the abdominal muscles and the womb. There are numerous reasons why it might be necessary, including: if the baby is in the breech position; if the placenta is covering the cervix; if the mother has pre-eclampsia or pregnancy-related high blood pressure; if the mother has genital herpes or untreated HIV; if there is excessive vaginal bleeding; if delivery needs to happen immediately because the baby is in danger; if it is twins or a multiple birth. Sometimes a woman will know during her pregnancy that she would prefer to have a baby by caesarean section on non-medical grounds: she might have endured previously traumatic births, mental ill-health, sexual abuse or violence.

The National Institute for Health and Care Excellence (NICE) issued guidelines in 2011 saying that a woman's choice about how to give birth should be respected by the NHS – but in 2018, an investigation by the childbirth charity Birthrights found that as many as three-quarters of NHS Trusts do not have written guidelines that clearly commit to upholding a woman's autonomy. Some NHS Trusts have implemented blanket policies that effectively ban maternal-request caesareans.[27]

It is a contentious subject: the World Health Organization's advice runs counter to the NICE guidelines. According to the WHO, caesarean sections should only be carried out when medically necessary as the surgical procedure can put the health of women and their babies at risk.[28]

In a culture where the bodies of women are undermined and under-researched, where our reproductive rights are controlled and curbed, it is to be expected that birth becomes a political issue, with opposing sides and controversial figures. But for pregnant women, that is unhelpful and distressing. Women should be trusted to make the best decisions for their bodies and their babies, after being given clear and impartial information and guidance.

Rebecca Schiller points out that it is necessary to research the reasons why the rate of caesarean sections is rising internationally (in Brazil, more than half of all births are C-sections)[29] but stresses that we must be careful not to conflate a global health issue with the human rights of the individual giving birth:

The caesarean birth rate is rising globally at such a high rate, and it has been shown that there are generally worse health outcomes for women and babies so there needs to

173

be a holistic assessment of why that is happening. But that should not become an argument about whether caesareans for individual women are good or bad – that's a very different argument. Many women feel that a caesarean birth would be best for them, for really excellent reasons, and they should be enabled to make that choice.

Women should be empowered to make the best decision for themselves. There is a notion, Schiller says, that if we start to 'allow' women to choose a C-section birth on non-medical grounds, there will be an alarming increase. This is, she argues, 'complete bullshit': 'I think most women would quite like to avoid major abdominal surgery. And for those women who've made a decision that, actually, that is best for them, they have some really compelling reasons.'

A significant majority of women will experience pregnancy and childbirth but, for each one of them, it will likely be one of the most momentous moments in their life. Giving birth is common but it is not straightforward – every day, throughout the world, 830 girls and women die in childbirth or from pregnancy complications. The majority of these deaths occur in developing countries: the maternal mortality ratio in the world's least developed countries is 436 deaths for every 100,000 live births.[30] In the UK the figure is 8.8.[31] In the US, the figure is 26[32] and the maternal mortality rate is rising, even as it declines in most other developing and developed countries.

We must demand that the international community does more to stop maternal death everywhere: we must ask how restricting the reproductive rights of girls and women contributes to preventable maternal death, and we must challenge the decline in global aid for maternal health.[33] We must address the role race plays in maternal mortality: in the US, black women are more than three times more likely to die from pregnancy-related causes as their white counterparts.[34] We must talk about birth, not as a homogenous occurrence but as a variable, individual event. To fully support women, we must educate ourselves about the realities of pregnancy and childbirth. We must re-educate ourselves, too, stripping away patriarchal assumptions and lazy generalizations.

After a woman gives birth it is essential that an honest and compassionate conversation continues. A lot will have changed for the new mother: she will be caring for a baby; she might be breastfeeding; if she had a C-section, she will be recovering from the operation; and if she gave birth vaginally, she is likely to be experiencing pain or discomfort.

Almost 90 per cent of women who give birth vaginally will have had tearing or an episiotomy. Pain is common, especially in the first month as the tear or cut heals and the stitches dissolve. One woman I speak to says:

> After the episiotomy, I couldn't sit for a month without being in extreme pain. Unfortunately this is when you have to sit constantly to breastfeed. Whenever my baby wasn't feeding, I had to lie on my side to take the weight off my vagina.

As women are often breastfeeding in this first month, pain relief options are limited to paracetamol or ibuprofen. 'It's insane given how big a procedure it is,' says one friend who had an episiotomy. 'Eventually [doctors] prescribed me some breastfeeding-friendly codeine for it, but they made me feel like I was overreacting.'

The pelvic floor muscles are likely to have come under strain during pregnancy and birth and weaker pelvic floor muscles make it harder to control the bowel and bladder. During the first four weeks after childbirth, around half of women experience urinary incontinence and as many as 10 per cent will experience faecal incontinence, especially if they had tears through the anal sphincter and rectum.[35]

Generally, doctors advise that penetrative sex is avoided for six weeks after birth, but some women I speak to have felt that they needed to wait much longer. Oestrogen levels are lower following birth, especially if a woman is breastfeeding, and this can cause vaginal dryness, which makes sex painful. 'No one tells you this!' says a friend who has recently become a mother. 'And lube did not help. Having sex for the first time after having the baby was like losing my virginity. I cried afterwards. I haven't had sex since.' Some women report that their vagina feels larger or that there's less sensation during sex after birth.

For most, the pain and incontinence and the discomfort will be temporary, subsiding in a few weeks or months. For some, though, symptoms will persist. A report in 2014 found that ten years after giving birth, around 20 per cent of mothers continue to experience urinary incontinence and around 3 per cent continue to experience faecal incontinence.[36] Around half of all women who have given birth will experience some degreee of pelvic prolapse, which involves the womb, bowel or bladder slipping from their normal position and bulging into the vagina, causing pain and discomfort.[37] These women will need support, working with specialist physiotherapists and gynaecologists. Sometimes women suffering from pain and incontinence will need mental health support.

In France, it is standard for all new mothers to be referred to a specialist physiotherapist who will work with them to strengthen their pelvic floor muscles, using a regime of exercises and electronic stimulation. In the UK, however, there is no tradition of automatic state-sponsored care for women and their vaginas after pregnancy. Actually, it can be common for new mothers to struggle to get a referral to see a physiotherapist or specialist.

In 2018, Mumsnet published a survey of 1224 British mothers as part of their campaign for better postnatal care. Thirty-four per cent of women said: 'I had a tear/injury but did not have adequate care and advice.' When asked 'If sex has become physically painful or uncomfortable as a result of giving birth, have you received any medical care focused on improving things for you?', just 4 per cent of women answered, 'I have received great medical care.' Eight per cent said: 'I have asked for medical care but have not had any.' Tellingly, 75 per cent of women answered: 'I have received no medical care and have not asked for any.' Vaginas and sex are still difficult to discuss in British culture – and that doesn't seem to improve even when a woman pushes a baby through her own vagina. Actually it might just get worse. There is a sense, perhaps, that a healthy baby is all that matters and a healthy vagina is a luxury, just like that C-section.

Speaking as the campaign was launched, the founder and CEO of Mumsnet, Justine Roberts, pointed out that some women's concerns were being dismissed because their problems didn't prevent penetrative sex. She said: 'Most enraging is the fact that we've seen some accounts of women who've approached healthcare professionals only to be told that mothers must expect everything to be different after birth, or "so long as your husband can penetrate you, it's fine". This is misogyny, pure and simple.'[38]

It is cruelly misogynistic, this disinterest in the vaginas of mothers, but as I interrogate new mums, I notice something hopeful. Even among those who have experienced pain and incontinence, there is a sense of wonder after birth at what the body – and the vagina – can do. 'You lose all sense of modesty. And the flipside of that is the pride in your body and what it has achieved,' says one woman.

Women who have looked in a mirror as they have given birth describe the experience as 'mind-blowing' and 'incredible'. One tells me:

> The way that the vagina changes and the way that it opens, is just staggering. I was really amazed at what felt like this miraculous thing that my body could do. It felt very powerful. It was the beginning of a more real relationship with my body, that wasn't about what other people thought of it, but actually, I know this thing that it can do. And I see it in my children every day, you know, I grew you and I pushed you out of there.

The pride women take in their own vaginas after giving birth shouldn't be secret – and neither should the pain they experience. Pregnancy, abortion, miscarriage and birth are common but extraordinary – each story is unique. Women benefit when those stories are told – and listened to.

# CHAPTER ELEVEN

# The Vagina and Menopause

*It is commonly thought that time is the particular enemy of women. Because we supposedly have so much to lose: our 'looks', our fertility, our cultural capital. There have been feminist modifications to this story over the years, but it remains powerful: a tale long told by men and subsequently retold and internalised by women.*

*But there are other ways of looking at it. That women have timepieces built into their bodies – primarily 'biological clocks' and the menopause – signs that must eventually be heeded, signs that are, finally, impossible to ignore, seems to me at least as much gift as curse.*

Zadie Smith, *Elle India*, May 2018

Suddenly, shamefully, I realize that I have never asked my mother about the menopause. We are close, I talk to her often, we can speak about most things. But when she experienced the menopause in her early fifties, around a decade ago, I overlooked it. I was in in my mid-twenties, a particularly selfish age I think, looking back on it, concerned with my (disastrous)

career and my (also disastrous) love life. I would sit around reading magazine articles about the notion of the quarter-life crisis
– being twenty-five is so hard, I would think – as my mother
consulted pamphlets she had picked up at the doctor's on the
menopause. Magazines, it seemed, were much more interested
in the imagined age-related issues of twenty-something women
than the genuine concerns of menopausal women.

Menopausal women have been missing from our culture,
from our films and TV shows. When 2000 Hollywood film
scripts were analysed in 2016, a huge disparity in the number
of lines spoken by male and female characters was discovered.
When actors were aged 22–31, men had 28 million words versus
women's 21 million. Aged 32–41, men had 44 million words versus women's 18 million (note how men are getting more verbose
as they get older, women less so). Aged 42–65, men had 55 million words: this was when they were most powerful, when they
delivered impassioned monologues or portrayed sparring law-
yers or wooed much younger women with long-winded jokes.
Aged 42–65, women had 11 million words. They were being
disappeared.[1]

In 2013, the UK TV industry faced accusations of sexism
and ageism when it was revealed that only 7 per cent of the TV
workforce, both on and off screen, were women over the age of
fifty.[2] High-profile female TV presenters spoke of being forced
out of jobs after they turned fifty. In 2015, a House of Lords
report concluded that the BBC had a policy of discriminating
against older women and covering it up with gagging orders.[3]

When menopausal women are missing from the mainstream
culture so is talk of menopause. If we rarely see the menopause depicted or discussed on TV or in movies, that silence
makes its way into our real lives, too, into workplaces, even into
families.

In the West, a woman's life is presented as a series of dead-lines, with particular focus on her early thirties, as society and biology's constraints conspire to create a pile-up of pressures: there should be an engagement by twenty-nine, marriage at thirty-one, a job that offers security and maternity leave by thirty-two, and don't forget the baby by thirty-five, whatever you do. I suppose that's why I was so concerned with my quarter-life crisis that day ten years ago. The deadline chat begins to fade away after a woman turns forty or so. The pressure is off but what comes next? Her lines are taken away from her, the cameras stop rolling.

Ten years too late, I phone my mother and ask her about the menopause. 'It was great,' she says. This enthusiasm should not surprise me. My mother is cheery. She is resilient. She keeps fit and weighs the same now as she did on her wedding day in the early 1980s. She has never had depression. I have only seen her ill a couple of times in my life. But, even so, in the rare instances I have heard the menopause discussed in the media or mentioned among colleagues, it has usually been in negative terms. And so I am dubious about this 'great'.

'Great?' I ask. 'Really?'

'Well, maybe I shouldn't say it's great,' she backtracks. 'It can be so bad for lots of people, and there are miserable things about it. But not having your period, after decades of period pain, really is great. It's great.'

Once I set out to educate myself about the menopause, I realize that my mother's position might not be so rare. I have seen that pregnancy and childbirth are specific to the individual, I have seen that arousal and orgasm are specific to the individual, I have seen that the hymen and the appearance of the vulva are specific to the individual. And I realize now that menopause is similar, affecting women in different ways. It is barely noticed by some and becomes a ten-year-long ordeal for others. When we don't talk about the menopause, we don't talk about its variability.

So, how can we define the menopause and talk about it in a way that feels relevant to and reflective of as many women as possible?

Some quick facts. Menopause is the time in a woman's life when she stops menstruating and can no longer get pregnant naturally. For women reaching menopause naturally (as opposed to a menopause due to medical treatment), it is defined as the day when a woman has not had a period for twelve consecutive months. Sometimes periods can stop abruptly but generally they start to become less frequent over months or years before they stop altogether. This time when periods are changing in frequency is known as perimenopause; the day when a woman has not had a period for twelve months is menopause; after that, she is post-menopausal. Generally, though, we use the term menopausal to refer to the time when there are symptoms.

Menopausal symptoms generally begin in the mid-forties and the average age to reach menopause in the UK is fifty-one. One in 100 women experience the menopause before they turn forty, one in 1000 women experience it before they turn thirty. Menopause before the age of forty is referred to as premature ovarian insufficiency (POI). In some rare cases, women do not reach menopause until their early sixties. Symptoms of the menopause do not have a clear beginning and ending; they may continue for a number of years after menopause.[4]

When I read about the symptoms of menopause I think back to my mother's cheery 'great'. So many of the possibilities associated with this period of mid-life sound brutal and harrowing.

I consult the NHS website and various books on the subject, I read personal accounts on online menopause forums and I talk to women who have experienced the menopause. On official websites (although not on the forums) the tone is often bright and upbeat, but there is no avoiding the fact that menopausal symptoms can be bleak, they can disrupt a woman's life – affecting her capacity to enjoy sex, to be able to work, to make it through the day without crying.

Weight gain is a symptom. A sudden onset or worsening of PMS symptoms might occur. A reduced or absent libido can be common. Insomnia. Breast pain. Mood swings, especially if a woman has been prone to PMS in the past. Memory problems, with fogginess and difficulty concentrating. Dry hair. Thin skin. Hairy skin. Acne. Worsening migraines. Recurring urinary tract infections and cystitis. Occasional heavy periods. Joint and muscle pain. Some women will find that depression, anxiety and panic attacks arise or worsen. There can be various changes in the vagina and vulva, including vaginal dryness and a thinning of the skin of the vagina and vulva, which might cause irritation, itching and soreness, especially during sex.

And then there are hot flushes, perhaps the most well-known symptom of menopause. 'Hot flushes' don't sound so bad but they can be incapacitating for some women. They are the most common symptom of the menopause, occurring in up to 80 per cent of women.[5] *Menopause: The Change for the Better*, a book compiled by Henpicked, an online community for women over forty, describes them like this:

> They usually come on very suddenly and spread through your body, chest, neck and face. They can vary in length from a few minutes to much longer. They can be associated with symptoms such as sweating, dizziness,

light-headedness and even heart palpitations. They can occur many times throughout the day and can continue for many years – some women experience hot flushes later in life, in their 70s and 80s.[6]

My mother remembers having the worst hot flushes in the peri-menopausal stage, when she was still working as a teacher:

> I would be sitting in front of thirty children and I'd feel the heat start suddenly at my feet and it would rush up my body. The children would look at me and say, 'Teacher, why is your face so red?' I was so flushed, burning up.

She felt flustered but it was manageable, she says.

In her book on the menopause – *The Change* – Germaine Greer addresses the variability in the severity of menopause symptoms, including hot flushes:

> Some women feel a sensation as if they had been sprayed with hot oil, which quickly passes and can be easily ignored. Others find that as a sensation of heat fades, they are seized by shivering and cold sweats; still others suffer palpitations, panic attacks or feel their skin crawling. At night the same dysfunction can cause disturbance of sleep and night sweats so copious that the sufferer must change her nightclothes and her bedding. Some women find that a hot flush can be expected after dealing with a crisis or making a concerted physical effort; others find the recurrence of flushing completely unpredictable.[7]

The duration and the severity of menopausal symptoms vary from woman to woman. Eight in ten women experience some menopausal symptoms, 25 per cent of women have severe symptoms. On average, most symptoms last around four years. However, around one in ten women experiences them for up to twelve years.[8]

If a woman experiences the menopause suddenly – for example if she receives cancer treatment to stop the body producing oestrogen because the hormone feeds breast and ovarian cancers; or if she has a hysterectomy or double oophorectomy – the symptoms might be worse.

Menopausal symptoms are caused by hormonal changes. Ovaries are the source of oestrogen and progesterone – the two key hormones that control the menstrual cycle and fertility in women. Oestrogen nourishes the tissues of the body with blood, including the vagina and skin. It regulates cholesterol and keeps organs like the brain, liver and heart healthy. Until menopause, it is mainly produced in the ovaries but, when ovulation stops, the fatty tissue, breast tissue, adrenals and liver take over, with lower levels produced. Progesterone helps control blood sugar levels and plays a crucial role in achieving and maintaining pregnancy. When ovulation stops, progesterone continues to be produced in the body, but at lower levels, too. Testosterone plays a key role in oestrogen production, supports bone density, helps turn fat into muscle, helps to improve cognitive function and contributes to libido. It declines with age. By menopause, the level of testosterone is at half of its peak, which occurs during a woman's twenties.

These hormonal shifts, as well as the general impact of ageing, will spell changes for the vulva, vagina and urethra. A decrease in oestrogen will mean that skin becomes drier and for many that affects the vagina and urethra, too.

Genitourinary syndrome of menopause (GSM) is a fairly new term, which doctors and menopause experts have been using since the mid-2010s. Previously called vulvovaginal atrophy, atrophic vaginitis or simply persistent vaginal dryness, it is a common symptom of the menopause, estimated to affect up to 50 per cent of women.[9]

The thinning and weakening of the tissues around the neck of the bladder and the urethra may prompt symptoms, such as a persistent or urgent need to urinate or recurring urinary tract infections and cystitis. Women often find that symptoms are passed off as unimportant or as an inevitability of ageing.

Greer writes:

What is true of GSM is also true of what is too often called 'sensitive bladder', which too is likely to remain untreated until the sufferer finds herself in aged care, by which time it may be too late. Meanwhile fortunes are made marketing incontinence pants, usually given a target audience of sedentary older women, on TV and well before the watershed. There is no public service ad that urges women to ask their doctor about 'overactive' or 'sensitive' bladder.[10]

When GSM affects the vagina, women might notice that the tissue of the vagina and vulva becomes thinner, drier and inflamed. There might be an itching or burning sensation. The vagina may shrink and become less likely to expand during sex, causing painful sex, often referred to as 'dyspareunia' by medics. It can feel like it is impossible to be penetrated. Recurring thrush can occur and pain and discomfort is likely even when a woman isn't sexually active or when she avoids penetrative sex.

Unlike many symptoms of menopause, GSM is chronic and unlikely to go away or get better with time. It is crucial then that women go to their doctor. Greer says there should be adverts on TV urging women to do so and experts tend to agree that there needs to be a proactive approach to treating GSM. It is a common condition that can cause great physical discomfort as well as emotional distress and mental ill-health. In one study of women with GSM, 17 per cent of women said it had negatively affected their self-esteem and 13 per cent said that it had negative consequences for their marriage.[11]

Too often, though, women who are experiencing significant pain and discomfort, women who are suffering emotional distress, don't do anything, don't know they *can* do anything. One study shows that approximately one-third of women with GSM do not go to a doctor with their symptoms.[12] Some women will look for over-the-counter relief and, while lubricants or vaginal moisturizers might help some, they will not work for everyone. There is a lack of information surrounding GSM and the treatments available, which leads to women suffering in silence.

In a survey carried out by the British Menopause Society in 2016, more than two in five women said that symptoms of the menopause had been worse than they had expected, but half said that they had not consulted a doctor as they felt the menopause was just something they had to 'put up with'.[13]

The survey prompted hand-wringing within the medical profession and a call for women experiencing menopausal symptoms to go to the GP, where they could expect clear and compassionate advice and treatments. Unfortunately, many women feel apathetic about seeking treatment; there is an inevitability to the symptoms, they suspect; an inevitability, too, to the response by doctors.

The novelist and memoirist Jeanette Winterson perfectly

describes the situation faced by women during mid-life in an essay about her own search for treatment for menopausal symptoms:

> A woman talks to her GP like a sinner at confession: 'It must be my hormones' covers everything from not wanting to sleep with your husband, to wanting to kill him. Meanwhile your waistline expands and your hair falls out. The prescription is likely to be the same: antidepressants or HRT.[14]

Hormonal replacement therapy (HRT) has, for more than half a century, been the most common treatment for the symptoms of menopause. But for almost as long, it has been caught up in controversy. Even today, how a woman feels about HRT is likely to be influenced by her relationship with her own GP or her views on the pharmaceutical industry or the newspapers and columnists she reads or any number of conflicting, contradictory and confusing factors.

Shortly after the contraceptive pill became widely available in the US in the early 1960s, the pharmaceutical industry introduced oestrogen replacements designed for use by women during the menopause. It was a great commercial success almost immediately, with millions of American women signing up. It was introduced in the UK in 1965 and proved popular here, too. Critics, including feminists opposed to the increasing medicalization of women's bodies, pointed out that women continued to produce oestrogen even after menopause, albeit less of it. They argued that the symptoms of the menopause faded after a few years, regardless of whether treatment was given. Their concerns were largely ignored, however, and by the mid-1970s, half of all post-menopausal women in the US were using HRT.[15]

Soon though, there was a noticeable increase in the cases of womb (endometrial) cancer and after the media reported the link, sales slowed.

Doctors discovered that by prescribing progesterone, or, more accurately, a synthetic steroid called progestogen that resembles it, they could counteract the harmful effects of the synthetic oestrogen. Basically, oestrogen encouraged an over-growth of the lining of the womb, which could cause womb cancer, whereas progesterone regulated the endometrium. Once this was discovered, women who were taking oestrogen were also advised to take progesterone, unless they had had a hyster-ectomy, which meant there was no risk of womb cancer.

Throughout the 1980s and 1990s menopausal women con-tinued to take HRT to alleviate their symptoms, but two major studies around the turn of the millennium raised fresh concerns. A study called the Women's Health Initiative, which examined the health effects on tens of thousands of women taking either oestrogen-only HRT or combined HRT, compared to women taking an identical placebo, began in the US in 1993.[16] As it became clear that the study was indicating that HRT increased the risks of coronary heart disease, invasive breast cancer, stroke and deep vein thrombosis, one arm of the study was dropped. The dramatic cancellation led to sensational headlines and con-fusion among doctors and their patients. The Million Women Study, which collected questionnaires on HRT use and its effects on certain issues of women's health, had begun in the UK in 1996 and, in 2003, it consolidated the panic by releasing its find-ing that there was a link between the use of HRT and a higher risk of breast cancer.[17]

Both studies were criticized at the time, with experts pointing out the shortcomings and flaws in the processes, but while the sci-ence was complicated, the headlines weren't. Amid safety fears, the number of women using HRT in the UK between 2003 and 2007 halved, falling from two million to less than one million.[18]

In 2015, NICE released its first-ever guidelines on menopause, advising that doctors give women clear information on HRT and recommending it for the treatment of hot flushes, night sweats and other symptoms of the menopause.[19] It was estimated at the time that the NICE advice could mean that the number of women taking HRT would double once again, increasing to two million.[20]

In 2017, the Women's Health Initiative, which had continued after the 2002 controversy, released research findings that showed taking HRT pills had no effect on life expectancy.[21] 'Hormone replacement therapy (HRT), possibly the most controversial medicine ever invented, will not kill you,' reported the *Guardian* at the time.[22]

There is more clarity about HRT, and the advantages and disadvantages, now than perhaps there has been at any point previously, but it's unsurprising that women still feel confused. 'I think I'd rather stick with my symptoms than get breast cancer,' one woman I speak to tells me. It's a misunderstanding of the risks – but it isn't difficult to see why she feels so unsure.

As well as HRT pills, there are now patches and gels. Oestrogen tablets can be inserted into the vagina to help reduce the symptoms of GSM. Unless women have had a hysterectomy, they will likely be prescribed progestogen, too. Testosterone can be prescribed if low levels are detected, which can improve mood, libido and energy levels.

Some women will be lucky to see a GP who is knowledgeable about the menopause or they will be referred to a menopause expert; others will find that they have to do a lot of the research themselves, educating themselves and re-educating themselves.

\*

In the UK, women who can afford private treatment and feel let down by the NHS and HRT might seek alternatives. Bioidentical hormones are thought by some to be safer and more effective than other types of HRT because they are more 'natural'. Oprah Winfrey and Kim Cattrall have spoken about the benefits of bioidenticals and Jeanette Winterson writes: 'Bio-identicals are made from plant sources – usually wild yams or soya beans, and because they have an identical structure to the hormones our bodies produce, our bodies tolerate them.'[23]

The NHS is emphatically opposed to bioidenticals, however, stating: 'Several remedies (such as bioidentical hormones) are claimed to help with menopausal symptoms, but these aren't recommended because it's not clear how safe and effective they are.'[24]

'Vaginal rejuvenation' is another much-maligned treatment sometimes used by women experiencing menopausal symptoms, particularly vaginal dryness and urinary incontinence. The name is off-putting and so is the fact that vaginal rejuvenation generally involves lasers or other energy-based devices. The FDA is clear in its condemnation, stating in 2018 that: 'These products have serious risks and don't have adequate evidence to support their use for [symptoms relating to the menopause]. We are deeply concerned women are being harmed.'[25]

That seems unequivocal, but I feel conflicted when I speak to Dr Jacqueline Lewis, the plastic surgeon from Chapter 6, who regularly carries out vaginal rejuvenation on 'women who have dry vaginas, either post-menopause or post-chemotherapy, or because they are on anti-hormone treatment'.

Dr Lewis explains that sometimes she sees patients who cannot be prescribed oestrogen for vaginal dryness because it would feed their breast or ovarian cancer:

I treat breast cancer patients who often are put into the menopause at a very young age after chemo, and they used to say, 'What can I do for the vaginal dryness?' And some of them were oestrogen-receptor-positive, which meant I couldn't give them oestrogen for their dryness, and I used to say, 'Yeah, just use lots of KY Jelly.' And there was one woman in particular, who said, 'I've practically used up the whole KY Jelly supply in Chiswick – is there nothing more because it doesn't really work?'

After learning about vaginal rejuvenation at a conference, Dr Lewis began offering it to her patients. 'I condemn people who make money out of vulnerable women and their insecurities,' she says. 'But there is something to be said about offering these treatments to the right person at the right time.'

It is easy to detect a sniffiness around expensive treatments for symptoms of the menopause. Of course, we must ensure that women are safe – that should always be paramount – but we should watch out for shades of, 'Oh these ridiculous women and their luxury vaginas.'

After decades of conflicting advice, dramatic headlines, overlooked pain and misunderstood symptoms, I don't think that it is unreasonable that women want to investigate treatments that go beyond incontinence pads, a bottle of lube and mini fans. I don't think that it is unreasonable that women have doubts about HRT.

There is an increasing openness about menopause, you can sense it. TV presenters and actresses who have been allowed to stick around past fifty are inclined to bring it up. Menopause is not the only thing a woman over fifty will want to talk about;

it might be the last thing a woman over fifty will want to talk about. But when women have lines and roles as they enter middle age, when they stay centre-stage, rather than being written out and written off, the menopause can become a subject for discussion and art and entertainment. And it needn't be funny. There has been a tendency for the menopause to be discussed only in comedic terms, as if laughing at hot flushes or vaginal dryness is the only way to discuss the issue. As Aminatou Sow, who went through an early menopause after surgery to treat womb cancer, says: 'It is always a punchline, right. You're always supposed to laugh at this stuff. And I'm like, let me tell you, this is not funny.'[26] When more menopausal women are actually writing the scripts, it's pretty likely that there will be fewer lame jokes.

The shift in how we talk about the menopause is happening slowly. For now, problems persist. A recent study found that a quarter of women have considered leaving their job because of symptoms of the menopause.[27] Ageism and misogyny combine to create workplaces in which women feel unsupported or humiliated. Hot flushes can feel mortifying in an office environment that is dismissive or mocking. A constant urge to pee might feel impossible to manage in an office building where there are not enough toilets. When employers are considering introducing menstrual leave policies, they must also consider menopause policies.

Silence has bred ignorance. And there must be a concerted effort to counteract that. A menopause re-education shouldn't just involve women over forty-five or specialist doctors. It needs to involve employers, designers, architects, movie producers, writers, policy makers, partners, daughters, sons. It needs to involve ideas and invention and ingenuity. Perhaps, most importantly, it needs to involve compassion.

A woman experiencing menopause might find renewed energy and freedom. She might look at all she has achieved, with her body and her mind and soul, and she might think, *Great.* She might consider all the time that is still to come, without worrying about pregnancy and period pain and infant children, and she might think, *Great.* But there might be days and weeks and months and even years when it is not so great. In greatness and not-so-greatness, women experiencing menopause should feel supported and represented.

# CHAPTER TWELVE

# Does My Vagina
# Define Me?

*Before I get to the city, street, house or bedroom I live in,
I spend more time in my body than anywhere else, and if
that's not right then I can't do much else.*

Juliet Jacques, *Trans: A Memoir*

Over tens of thousands of words, I have argued that we should all be much more open, much more honest, much more vocal about our vaginas and our vulvas and our genitals generally. However, as soon as I begin to look at the trans experience, I realize that this isn't necessarily an option that is available to or practical for the trans community. There is a prurient curiosity about the bodies, and the genitals, of trans people, one that has been facilitated by the media's before-and-after narratives.

Janet Mock, the US author of the bestselling memoir *Redefining Realness: My path to womanhood, identity, love & so much more*, put it this way in 2014: 'I don't talk about my kitty cat with my friends... But I – an unapologetic trans woman and writer – have been asked about my vagina (by people I do not know, mind you) more times than I can even recall.'[1]

People are nosy about the genitals of trans people; people are derisive about the genitals of trans people, as if, simply by being trans, a person has invited speculation and even cruelty about their body. A reluctance to discuss vaginas or genitalia is utterly understandable in the face of such invasiveness. When living in a culture that fetishizes their genitals, that *focuses* on their genitals, many trans people feel safer and happier not talking about their genitals.

There is a horrible bit (actually, the whole thing is horrible – don't watch it) in Ricky Gervais's Netflix comedy special, *Humanity*, where he talks about Caitlyn Jenner, who is probably the most well-known trans woman in America. Gervais giggles like a strange, giddy child when he imagines Jenner going to the doctor to request genital surgery. There's a glee in Gervais's eyes as he affects a deep voice and mimes a penis. I've watched it twice now – the first time I didn't know what to expect, I was just browsing Netflix on my sofa on a cold, dark evening; the second time I did it to take notes. Both times, I felt not just not entertained but actually sad and disquieted. It's unsavoury and unedifying, this puerile joke performed by a man high on his imagined sense of transgressiveness. 'I can't say it, I can't say it,' his grin seems to suggest but the thing is he *can* say it – and he *is* saying it. He is saying it in front of thousands of his fans and they all laugh whenever he gives them any signal to laugh, so suddenly there are all these laughs and whoops and giggles and cheers, reverberating around this theatre, all directed towards Caitlyn Jenner and her body – and her genitals, in particular.

It is upsetting to watch, bleak and grimy-feeling. It must be worse, much worse, if you are trans.

*

Stonewall, the UK charity that fights for lesbian, gay, bi and trans equality, defines trans as:

> An umbrella term to describe people whose gender is not the same as, or does not sit comfortably with, the sex they were assigned at birth. Trans people may describe themselves using one or more of a wide variety of terms, including (but not limited to) transgender, transsexual, gender-queer (GQ), gender-fluid, non-binary, gender-variant, crossdresser, genderless, agender, nongender, third gender, two-spirit, bi-gender, trans man, trans woman, trans masculine, trans feminine and neutrois.[2]

CN Lester, the author of *Trans Like Me*, puts it this way:

> Any person who has had to challenge or change the sexed and gendered labels placed upon them at birth to honour their true selves can, by their own or others' volition, find themselves under this trans umbrella. The category of trans can be an uncomfortable place to be, filled with the fears society has about disruption, fitting in, danger and change.[3]

The reason I bring up the trans experience here, in this book about vaginas, is because when we recognize trans rights, trans lives and the validity of trans identities, we recognize that not all girls and women have a vagina and that not everyone who has a vagina is a girl or a woman.

Some, but not all, trans people have gender dysphoria, meaning that they experience discomfort or distress because there is a mismatch between their sex assigned at birth and their gender identity. A roughly equal number of boys and girls are thought to experience gender dysphoria, with the numbers seeking treatment in the UK growing every year, as awareness increases.[4] When it comes to adults, there is a serious lack of data about trans people so it is difficult to say very much about demographics – in 2018 the UK government said it didn't know how many trans people there were in the country and gave an estimate of 200,000 to 500,000.[5]

What feels certain is that trans women are more visible than other trans people in the media. There are probably several reasons for this. The fact that trans women are more visible in everyday life plays a part – trans men are often not recognized as trans, whereas trans women, especially if they are tall, often are. There is also more discussion, particularly in the UK, about the rights of trans women in relation to their access to single-sex spaces, particularly those designed to protect a disadvantaged group – women's shelters, for example. I think it's true to say, too, that in a patriarchy, there is more salacious interest in the bodies and sex lives of women and there is more interest in the appearance of women. *Time* magazine and *Vanity Fair* put Laverne Cox and Caitlyn Jenner on their covers, and the mainstream websites and TV channels follow their lead. Images of thin, glossy-haired, rich women, trans or cis, sell magazines and newspapers and generate clicks.

Among cis people, there can sometimes be an assumption, that to be trans means to have, or plan to have, gender-confirmation surgery, which is also known as sex-reassignment surgery. But this is not true for all trans people, perhaps not even for a majority. Again, it's difficult to get the data, but in one US study, 61 per cent of trans respondents reported having medically transitioned while 33 per cent said they had surgically transitioned. That same study showed that around 14 per cent of trans women and 72 per cent of trans men said they don't ever want full gender-confirmation surgery.[6] In UK law, there is no requirement for trans people to have surgery to be recognized as trans.

To 'transition' can mean to have gender-confirmation surgery. It can mean to medically transition – to use HRT, either oestrogen (a feminizing hormone) or testosterone (a masculinizing hormone). In young people, gonadotropin-releasing hormone (GnRH) analogues, which temporarily prevent the onset of hormones and block puberty, can be used. Transitioning can also involve laser hair removal, cosmetic surgery, the changing of pronouns and names, and top surgery, either breast augmentation or mastectomy.

Gender-confirmation surgery is sometimes called lower or bottom surgery and, in the UK, irreversible genital surgeries are not usually undertaken until a person is at least eighteen years old and has lived in the gender role that reflects their gender identity for more than twelve months.

For trans men, lower surgery is usually done in stages: some people will have just one or two procedures done; others will have several operations, depending on their desired outcome. There are sacrifices – a hysterectomy and oophorectomy will result in infertility so some trans men wait until after they've had children to proceed. And beyond that, there will be risks of loss of sexual sensation and risks of infection – the more complex the proposed surgery, the more risks there are. Lower surgery for trans women can generally be undertaken with fewer surgeries, sometimes just one procedure. Like with trans men, the decision to undergo surgery will depend on the individual, who can weigh up the risks and the sacrifices.

As a cis person, happy with her own genitals, the thought of surgery is daunting, but regrets after lower surgery are extremely rare: a 2008 UK study found that 98 per cent of those who had undergone genital gender-confirmation surgery were satisfied with the outcome.[7]

Lower surgery can make it easier for trans people to fit in in certain situations and, for some people, this is a priority. A trans woman I speak to puts it like this: 'Without a vagina, there are things that I can't do, like go swimming or try on certain clothes or just be next-to-naked in women's spaces.' Many other trans people, however, will find that living with genitalia that does not reflect their gender identity is possible, even preferable.

One trans woman, who I'll call Ani, tells me that she has had HRT and top surgery but hasn't had lower surgery because:

> My gender dysphoria ends around my bosom. With everything bust up, I can have intense days – I cover mirrors, I can't look at myself. It feels bizarre, it feels quite weird, I don't like seeing that at all. But downstairs, no, not at all.

Of course, she understands that other trans women might wish to have gender-confirmation surgery, but she wants us to question the assumption that to be a woman is to have a vagina. There has been a preoccupation in medicine, she feels, for doctors to operate according to their own biases. 'The way I see it is that we had a bunch of really sexist cisgender male doctors and they felt that one could medicalize transness by making the trans female body as close to the cisgender female body as possible.'

Sometimes surgery can, Ani says, play into 'patriarchal notions of femininity':

> It's awkward, because I think the public do perceive that the ultimate goal is to have gender-confirmation surgery, and then, you know, you're a real woman. For me, it's

very awkward to say this, but my arrival at womanhood was completely spiritual, it had nothing to do with the outside.

Of course, I've got dysphoria and, you know, it's very much been allayed by the HRT and the surgeries I've had, I can't deny that. But I've also had to accept that surgery has not increased my understanding of myself as a woman. That was just an absolute certainty from the age of three – I just see it as a neurological thing. Every time I was told that I wasn't a girl, wasn't a woman, it was just bizarre to me. I thought it was so weird. I thought, what are you talking about? It's crazy. I remember seeing my younger sister, who is cisgender, having her nappy changed, and looking at it and thinking, that's interesting, that's different. But it wasn't, 'Oh, I want that.' I just thought, 'Oh that's different, we are different.'

Ani finds new names for her genitals: 'My back passage was always a "pussy". And then there are names like "lady-stick" and "shenis" – it's quite hilarious really.'

Buck Angel is a trans porn producer and actor as well as a motivational speaker. In a 2018 essay titled 'How Learning to Love My Vagina Affirmed My Manhood', he explored the process in which he decided against lower surgery. It was painful, he explains, to feel 'like a freak of nature' but he slowly began to 'accept his vagina'.

He writes:

We don't speak positively about sex in the trans community. We shut it down, because of years of being told that genitals equal gender; years of feeling like the whole world is only focused on trans people's genitals, and that if we're open about our bodies, we'll be fetishized for it. I find that silence so incredibly damaging.

If we are open about sex, about our bodies, about the ways that we experience pleasure, we can help each other reach new levels of authenticity.[8]

Juno Roche, a writer, campaigner and founder of Trans Workers UK and the Trans Teachers Network, has written about life after lower surgery, observing that while she had thought it would 'answer all of the questions that had floated around my messy head for many years' that's not how it feels now:

> Over the past few years I've found truth and life in my wonkily queer body. I exist in my wonderful trans-ness. My neo-pussy isn't a cis vagina. No, to me it is far more elegant and multifarious than any simple copy or simulation.[9]

What is right for Ani and for Angel and for Roche won't be right for every trans person, of course. The decision to have or not to have lower surgery is deeply personal; so too is the decision to discuss your own genitals. Trans people don't owe us stories; they shouldn't *have* to tell us stories.

None of us should *have* to tell stories to get access to better legal or healthcare systems. We shouldn't have to tell stories about our urinary incontinence for employers to implement fairer and kinder menopause policies. We shouldn't have to tell stories about being sexually assaulted before universities and governments change guidelines and laws about harassment and rape. Sometimes, though, telling stories can be a powerful tool: during the Repeal The Eighth campaign ahead of the referendum on abortion in the Republic of Ireland in 2018, thousands of women shared their stories about having to travel to the UK and other parts of Europe to access abortion. The stories were moving, disturbing and effective – in one poll, more than 60 per cent said that hearing personal testimony was the single biggest factor in deciding how they would vote.[10] On 25 May 2018, Ireland voted by a landslide to legalize abortion.

And still: nobody should feel compelled to tell stories about their sexual and reproductive health. It should not be the only way to gain human rights.

When I have spoken to people about their genitals for this book, many people have told me personal and private information before quickly adding: 'You won't include my name, will you?' People don't want other people to know about their vaginal dryness or their abortion or about the details of how they gave birth. That's understandable: they want privacy and they don't want to feel that a stranger defines them by a single story about their genitals. Trans people share those concerns, but they must also consider their safety. Because when a trans person shares a story about their genitals they are likely to face hate and discrimination. Just to exist as a trans person often means facing hate and discrimination.

In 2017, a British survey found that more than one-third of trans people had been discriminated against because of their gender identity when visiting a café, restaurant, bar or nightclub within the last year.[11] Trans people are often rejected from their own families, leading to homelessness and mental ill-health – LGBTQ+ young people are more likely to be homeless than their non-LGBTQ+ peers and 69 per cent of LGBTQ+ homeless youth are highly likely to have experienced familial rejection, abuse and violence.[12] Black and minority ethnic (BAME) trans people are more likely to face discrimination on the basis of their race and gender and often their religion, too.[13]

There is sometimes a sense that to be a feminist who cares about vaginas is to be a person who does not care about trans rights. I reject this notion completely. To put it plainly, I think the suggestion that a woman can't care about vaginas *and* trans rights is deeply misogynistic.

In April 2018, Janelle Monáe released 'Pynk', a sweet-sounding but deeply empowering ode to the vagina. The lyrics were loaded with innuendo – the song opened 'Pink like the inside of your, baby / Pink behind all of the doors, crazy' – while the video was unequivocal. Monáe and a crew of black female dancers (including the actress Tessa Thompson) arrived in a pink-hued desert valley driving a pink convertible. They sat around the 'Pynk rest inn', clicking their fingers to the music, and then... well, then they lined up in a formation and it became obvious that five of them – including Monáe – were wearing pink pants that resembled the vulva, with the space between their knees representing the vaginal opening and the billowing folds of pink fabric representing the labia. In the dance sequence, a human head (Thompson's) was used to represent the clitoris.

Immediately, the song and video were rightfully praised as a celebration of black women and queer sexuality. Soon though, there were accusations that the video aligned itself with 'vagina-centric' feminism, which generally (or online at least) refers to feminism that places too much emphasis on biological sex and excludes women without vaginas. Monáe herself said on Twitter that 'Pynk' was celebrating women 'no matter if you have a vagina or not',[14] while Thompson tweeted: 'to all the black girls that need a monologue that don't have Vaginas, I'm listening'.[15]

One journalist at a women's site gave the video the thumbs up for celebrating black women and queerness, but not before she asserted that:

… pussy-centric feminism is rightly derided as cis-sexist, reductionist, and simply tired. Relying on the notion that 'women are united by their vaginas' is a shallow and basic reading that centers white cisgender women.[16]

It was not the first time women who have created art about vaginas have been disparaged. In 2016, *Vice* called Eve Ensler's *The Vagina Monologues* a 'play that empowered suburban moms across America', accusing it of being 'dated in a loveable Phoebe-from-Friends kind of way'.[17] It was a depressingly arrogant dismissal of a hugely significant project.

I think we can do better than this. I think we must do better than this. Making art or staging a protest about a crucial aspect of women's rights does not mean that we are denying other aspects of women's or marginalized people's rights. Vaginas and vulvas are not just a concern for privileged women, some unseen 'suburban' or 'white feminist' woman. All around the world, in suburbs, in cities, in villages, in prison, in homes, in schools, there are women who are abused or hurt or mutilated because they have a vagina and a vulva. Belittling feminism that involves the vagina and the vulva risks further stigmatizing the vagina and the vulva, risks allowing that hurt to continue.

I am a woman but I have not gone through childbirth. I know that this does not make me any less of a woman. Likewise, I know that ovaries or a vagina are not an essential component of womanhood. I know that a trans woman is a woman. I know that a man can have a vagina.

I also know that cis women's bodies are used to oppress them, I know that women face discrimination because they menstruate, because they get pregnant, because they experience the menopause. And so, I know that when a major international pop star, like Janelle Monáe, dresses up as a vulva it feels significant.

I want my feminism to work for trans women and recognize the specific and intersecting challenges women of colour and disabled women face. I want my feminism to acknowledge the ways in which capitalism and racism and strict gender roles work alongside misogyny to oppress women. I also want there to be room for us to discuss vaginas without being called 'basic'.

I do not believe that there has to be a battle between those who care about vaginas and those who care about trans rights. I think it is possible to care about both. There will be difficult conversations and learning curves and debate – but there does not have to be hate and disparagement.

Sometimes, the term 'people with cervixes' is used instead of 'women' in cervical-screening campaigns and pamphlets. The term is used so that non-binary people and trans men are not excluded from the process. I don't think that the term works, largely because I worry that not everyone who reads 'people with cervixes' will understand what it means. I would rather we used 'women *and* people with cervixes'. Maybe I am wrong. Maybe there is another option. I don't know. I'm learning. Most of us are. I would like to talk about it. And I would like to talk about it without my desire to talk about it being interpreted as a sign that I wish to undermine trans rights or align myself with people who do.

This 'people with cervixes' point is the sort of point that would be difficult to raise on Twitter because the platform, and the Internet in general, is unsympathetic to people who haven't *already* made up their mind. Certain corners of the Internet are interested in 'schooling' people but are often not equipped for genuine teaching and learning. The Internet can be deeply uncivil – and with conversation around gender, sex, genitals and human rights, we should be aiming for more than civility. We should be aiming for compassion and empathy. Social media hasn't been up to the job. The mainstream media hasn't been up to the job. Education can help get us there, I hope.

When we acknowledge the lives and rights of trans people in our education and re-education about the vagina, we will learn that trans people face specific challenges. Getting a period or going for a cervical screening as a trans man can intensify feelings of gender dysphoria. Learning that and recognizing that doesn't mean that I care any less about the vaginas, the periods and the cervical screenings of cis women.

An education that recognizes that gender isn't binary but a spectrum must also acknowledge that sex isn't always binary.

We are taught that chromosomes determine genitals, which determine sex, which determines gender. A sperm contains 22 chromosomes plus either an X or Y chromosome and meets an egg, which has 22 chromosomes plus an X chromosome. 46XX means it's a girl with a vagina and 46XY means it's a boy with a penis. But sometimes it's not that simple. Sometimes an egg or sperm may lack a sex chromosome or have an extra one so an embryo could be 45X or 45Y or 47XXY or 47XYY or 47XXX. And sometimes babies are born with both female and male anatomy, a vagina and testes, say, or a penis and ovaries.

As seen in Chapter 2, up to 1.7 per cent of people have some intersex traits, meaning they are born with sex characteristics – genitals, reproductive organs, chromosomal patterns – that do not neatly align with typical binary notions of female and male bodies. It is extremely rare for a baby to be registered as intersex, but extrapolating from World Health Organization figures,[18] it would appear that at least three babies a week are born with genital anomalies in the UK. Some intersex people or people with disorders of sex development (DSD) identify as trans; most do not.

Although intersex people (who were called hermaphrodites before campaigners pointed out that the term is confusing and stigmatizing) have pretty much always faced discrimination, it wasn't until relatively recently that they were *disappeared*. Since the 1930s, doctors in the West have operated on babies born with ambiguous genitalia, often in the first week of their lives. Parents who have intersex babies are told not to announce the birth until doctors have assigned a sex following an investigation and surgery. Sometimes surgery is necessary for the health of the baby, but in recent years there have been suggestions that unnecessary surgery on infants in an attempt to 'normalize' their genitalia is cruel and even a human-rights violation. The science of intersex variations is complicated and the reality of intersex life is often taboo but any humane, respectful and honest education about what it means to have genitals must aim to involve intersex people and their experience.

Around a year ago, I was really angry, I was furious about something that had happened at work. I spoke to an acquaintance, I told her about this rage that was travelling up through my body, barely controlled. 'You're probably getting your period,' she said. She recommended an app that could track my menstrual cycle and send me updates on expected moods; it could even, she said, send updates to my husband so that he could be aware if an oestrogen fluctuation was about to prompt a spell of fury.

I became more enraged. 'I am angry about work,' I said. 'I am angry about something that has happened at work.' I did not say it but I wanted to say: 'I am not angry because of my hormones or my ovaries or my vagina. I am not defined by my hormones or my ovaries or my vagina.'

I know that PMS is a genuine condition. I get PMS most months. Maybe that day, I even *had* PMS. But there was something about the way that she recommended the app – especially, I suppose, her suggestion that my husband could monitor my moods – that made me feel angrier, more furious.

Sometimes, I feel trapped by the idea of being a woman, by the idea that my anger is less palatable than a man's.

Sometimes I feel trapped by the biology of being a woman, by the blood I bleed each month.

Sometimes I feel trapped by the idea of the biology of being a woman, by the suggestion that my justified anger is not actually justified but a predictable reaction to a hormonal change, which precedes the blood that I bleed each month.

In *We Should All Be Feminists*, Chimamanda Ngozi Adichie addressed the way in which strict gender roles hold us all back, every single one of us, whatever our gender. She spoke of an anger she feels when she sees children being let down by a patriarchy that promotes unyielding ideas of what masculinity and femininity mean:

> I am angry. Gender as it functions today is a grave injustice. We should all be angry. Anger has a long history of bringing about positive change; but, in addition to being angry, I'm also hopeful. Because I believe deeply in the ability of human beings to make and remake themselves for the better.[19]

I am more than my vagina. I am more than my ovaries. I need to and I want to know about my vagina and my ovaries and my sexual and reproductive health. I need to and I want to know about my hormones. But I am more than that. I am more than a fluctuation in oestrogen. I am more than an angry woman. We are all more than our genitals and our gender. We all deserve a life that is not defined by our genitals and our gender. Let's stay furious until society recognizes that.

Let's talk. Let's hope. Let's make. Let's remake. Let's educate. Let's re-educate.

# Acknowledgements

Thank you to my agents Daisy Parente and Jane Finigan for their support, insight, guidance, wisdom and kindness. Thank you for believing in this project, and in me, from the earliest days.

Thank you to Clare Drysdale, an editor who understood this book from the start, who is calm and can-do, who is smart and generous, whose guidance and support was always felt.

Thank you to everyone at Allen & Unwin – especially to Carmen Rodriguez Balit and Kirsty Doole. Thank you to Julia Kellaway, for her shrewd and intelligent copy editing.

Thank you to the many women who provided invaluable insight, including Nimko Ali, Rebecca Schiller, Rachael Revesz, Rowan Ellis, Lucy Emmerson, Miss Adeola Olaitan, Professor Geeta Nargund, Mrs Jacqueline Lewis, Shelby Hadden, Jessica Hepburn and Bex Baxter.

Thank you Dr Grace Waxman and Charlie Alderwick for being early readers.

I am proud to have been a founding member of The Pool and over the years, it is there that I first became interested in, and started working on, so many of the stories I tell in this book.

To everyone who shared stories about their own bodies, some of whom would rather not be named: thank you.

Thank you to the ones who shared stories about their own vaginas or were early readers or kept me buoyant via Whatsapp messages or did all of those things. Thank you Niamh O'Keeffe, Katie Gibbons, India Whisker, Niamh Mulvey, Áine Lavin, Fiona O'Keeffe, Jean Hannah Edelstein, Deirdre Cole, Elizabeth Geary Keohane, Eimear Walsh, Lara Hickey, Hattie Crisell, Harriet Walker, Kelly Bowerbank, Liz Haycroft, Marisa Bate, Grace Banks and Rasha Kahil.

Thank you to my wonderfully supportive parents, Ann and Bill, and my funny, open and honest sisters, Ailbhe and Daire.

Thank you to the NHS and to the staff of Homerton University Hospital, in particular, who know a lot about my vagina and carry out crucial, important work every single day.

Thank you especially to Ben. For everything. It is an honour to face down challenges by your side. Your resilience is inspirational and your kindness is unending.

# Resources

Throughout this book, I have focused on areas where I thought that information has been particularly lacking but there is more, much more, to learn. There is more to discuss, there are more stories to tell, from different viewpoints, with different beginnings and endings. I hope that this is just the start of your re-education.

Below are resources I found helpful while writing this book, which I hope will be helpful for you, too.

*Reading List*

*An Excellent Choice*, Emma Brockes, Faber & Faber, 2018
*Bad Feminist*, Roxane Gay, Corsair, 2014
*Come As You Are*, Emily Nagoski, Scribe UK, 2015
*Dance Nation (Oberon Modern Plays)*, Clare Barron, Oberon Books Ltd, 2018
*Episiotomy: Physical and emotional aspects*, Sheila Kitzinger, National Childbirth Trust, 1981
*Everywoman: A gynaecological guide for life*, Derek Llewellyn-Jones, Penguin Life, 2015

*Fruit of Knowledge: The vulva vs the patriarchy*,
 Liv Strömquist, Virago, 2018
*Girls & Sex*, Peggy Orenstein, Oneworld Publications, 2016
*Giving Up the Ghost*, Hilary Mantel, Fourth Estate, 2010
*Headscarves and Hymens: Why the Middle East needs a sexual
 revolution*, Mona Eltahawy, Weidenfeld & Nicolson, 2016
*Outrageous Acts and Everyday Rebellions*, Gloria Steinem,
 Flamingo, 1985
*Testosterone Rex: Unmaking the myths of our gendered minds*,
 Cordelia Fine, Icon Books, 2017
*The Argonauts*, Maggie Nelson, Melville House UK, 2016
*The Change*, Germaine Greer, Bloomsbury, 2018
*The Empathy Exams: Essays*, Leslie Jamison, Granta Books,
 2015
*The Feminine Mystique*, Betty Friedan, Penguin Classics, 2010
*The Hidden Face of Eve: Women in the Arab world*, Nawal El
 Saadawi, Zed Books, 2015
*The Second Sex*, Simone de Beauvoir, Vintage Classics, 1997
*The Vagina Monologues*, Eve Ensler, Virago, 2018
*The Wonder Down Under: A user's guide to the vagina*, Dr Nina
 Brochmann and Ellen Stokken Dahl, Yellow Kite, 2018
*Trans: A Memoir*, Juliet Jacques, Verso, 2016
*Trans Like Me: A journey for all of us*, CN Lester, Virago, 2017
*Vagina: A new biography*, Naomi Wolf, Virago, 2013
*Why Human Rights in Childbirth Matter*, Rebecca Schiller,
 Pinter & Martin Ltd, 2016

### TV Shows, Films and Videos

'Cliteracy', Sophia Wallace, TEDxSalford, July 2015
*Crazy Ex-Girlfriend*, Rachel Bloom and Aline Brosh McKenna,
 Netflix

*I Love Dick*, Jill Soloway, Amazon Studios
*Private Life*, Tamara Jenkins, Netflix
'Vagina Dispatches', Mona Chalabi and Mae Ryan,
    *The Guardian*
'We Should All Be Feminists', Chimamanda Ngozi Adichie,
    TedxEuston, April 2013


## Podcasts

'Call Your Girlfriend', Aminatou Sow and Ann Friedman
'The Guilty Feminist', Deborah Frances-White
'Where Should We Begin?', Esther Perel, Audible
*Woman's Hour*, The Menopause series, BBC Radio 4


## Instagram

Bloody Good Period (www.instagram.com/bloodygoodperiod)
I Had A Miscarriage (www.instagram.com/ihadamiscarriage)
The Vulva Gallery (www.instagram.com/the.vulva.gallery)
Women's Environmental Network (www.instagram.com/
    wen_uk)


## Websites

Endometriosis UK (www.endometriosis-uk.org)
Free Periods (www.freeperiods.org)
Gender Identity Research & Education Society (www.gires.
    org.uk)
National Institute for Health and Care Excellence (www.nice.
    org.uk)
NHS (www.nhs.uk)
Our Bodies Ourselves (www.ourbodiesourselves.org)

Slutever (www.slutever.com)
Tommy's (www.tommys.org)

# References

## Introduction

1. Ehrenreich, B. and English, D., 1973. *Witches, Midwives, and Nurses: A history of women healers.*
2. Ehrenreich, B. and English, D., 2010. *Witches, Midwives, & Nurses: A history of women healers.* The Feminist Press, CUNY.

## Chapter One: *A Sex Re-education*

1. https://plan-uk.org/file/
   plan-uk-break-the-barriers-report-032018pdf/
   download?token=Fs-HYP3v
2. https://assets.publishing.service.gov.uk/government/
   uploads/system/uploads/attachment_data/file/413178/
   Not_yet_good_enough_personal__social__health_and_economic_
   education_in_schools.pdf
3. https://www.legislation.gov.uk/ukpga/1988/9/section/28
4. https://www.huffingtonpost.com/2013/04/12/
   margaret-thatcher-anti-gay-speech_n_3071177.html
5. http://koreajoongangdaily.joins.com/news/article/article.
   aspx?aid=3045301
6. https://qz.com/1289137/south-korea-has-a-sex-education-
   problem-and-these-teachers-are-trying-to-fix-it/
7. https://www.vox.com/science-and-health/2017/6/30/15894750/
   teen-birth-rates-hit-all-time-low

8. http://thehill.com/opinion/healthcare/396534-teens-deserve-better-than-abstinence-only-sex-ed
9. https://www.buzzfeednews.com/article/andrewkaczynski/mike-pence-in-2002-condoms-are-a-very-very-poor-protection-a#.ih673ZNvp
10. Orenstein, P., 2016. *Girls & Sex: Navigating the complicated new landscape.* Oneworld Publications.
11. https://www.fpa.org.uk/news/uk-has-highest-teenage-birth-rates-western-europe
12. https://www.bmj.com/content/360/bmj.j5930
13. https://metro.co.uk/2015/08/18/being-too-embarrassed-to-say-vagina-is-putting-young-womens-health-at-risk-5348263/
14. http://seksonderje25e.nl/files/uploads/Sex%20under%20the%20age%2025%202017%20summary.pdf
15. Schalet, A.T., 2011. *Not Under My Roof: Parents, teens, and the culture of sex.* University of Chicago Press.
16. Orenstein, P., 2016. *Girls & Sex: Navigating the complicated new landscape.* Oneworld Publications.
17. Schalet, A.T., 2011. *Not Under My Roof: Parents, teens, and the culture of sex.* University of Chicago Press.
18. https://www.independent.co.uk/life-style/health-and-families/health-news/vagina-study-nearly-half-of-british-women-cannot-identify-vulva-cervix-a7219656.html
19. https://www.bbc.co.uk/news/health-40410459

## Chapter Two: *The Facts (If We Can Call Them That)*

1. https://www.vice.com/en_uk/article/exmjye/stop-calling-it-a-vagina
2. Freitag, B., 2004. *Sheela-na-gigs: Unravelling an enigma.* Routledge.
3. https://www.atlasobscura.com/articles/sheelanagig-map-ireland
4. http://www.who.int/genomics/gender/en/index1.html
5. Sartre, J-P., 1992. *Being and Nothingness: A phenomenology essay on ontology.* Simon & Schuster, 782.
6. https://www.independent.co.uk/life-style/health-and-families/vulva-normal-vagina-health-study-labiaplasty-surgery-a8424371.html
7. https://www.bustle.com/p/11-signs-you-might-have-a-tilted-uterus-51952
8. Kilchevsky, A., Vardi, Y., Lowenstein, L. and Gruenwald, I., 2012. Is the female G-spot truly a distinct anatomic entity?. *The Journal of Sexual Medicine, 9*(3), pp.719–26.

9. https://www.vogue.com/article/goop-jade-yoni-egg-lawsuit-gwyneth-paltrow-vaginal-pelvic-floor-health

10. Herbenick D, Fu TC, Arter J, Sanders SA, Dodge B. Women's experiences with genital touching, sexual pleasure, and orgasm: results from a US probability sample of women ages 18 to 94. *Journal of Sex & Marital Therapy.* 2017 Aug 8:1-2.

11. https://www.the-pool.com/health/wombs-etc/2018/3/Eve-Ensler-20-years-of-The-Vagina-Monologues

## Chapter Three: *The Hymen, a Useless Symbol*

1. https://www.thelocal.se/20091208/23720

2. Gray, Henry. *Anatomy of the Human Body.* Philadelphia: Lea & Febiger, 1918; Bartleby.com, 2000. www.bartleby.com/107/.

3. https://www.thelocal.se/20091208/23720

4. El Saadawi, N., 2007. *The Hidden Face of Eve: Women in the Arab world.* Zed Books.

5. Eltahawy, M., 2015. *Headscarves and Hymens: Why the Middle East needs a sexual revolution.* Farrar, Straus and Giroux.

6. El Saadawi, N., 2007. *The Hidden Face of Eve: Women in the Arab world.* Zed Books.

## Chapter Four: *The Clitoris, and How It's Ignored*

1. Wolf, N., 2012. *Vagina: A new biography.* Virago.

2. Galen, 1968. *On the Usefulness of the Parts of the Body.* Cornell University Press.

3. See images from the book at: https://www.metmuseum.org/art/collection/search/349377

4. Wolf, N., 2012. *Vagina: A new biography.* Virago.

5. Ibid.

6. Williamson, S. and Nowak, R., 1998. The truth about women. *New Scientist*, 159(2145), pp.34–5.

7. https://studylib.net/doc/8339689/anatomy-of-the-clitoris---journal-of-urology--the

8. Wolf, N., 2012. *Vagina: A new biography.* Virago.

9. https://www.smh.com.au/national/anatomy-of-a-revolution-20050908-gdm13b.html

10. https://www.theguardian.com/education/2016/aug/15/french-schools-3d-model-clitoris-sex-education

11. Kinsey, A.C., Pomeroy, W.B., Martin, C.E. and Gebhard, P.H., 1998. *Sexual Behavior in the Human Female*. Indiana University Press.

12. https://www.theguardian.com/global-development/2018/jul/26/first-fgm-prosecution-in-somalia-history-death-10-year-old-girl

13. https://data.unicef.org/topic/child-protection/female-genital-mutilation/#

14. http://www.who.int/reproductivehealth/topics/fgm/about/en/

15. https://www.channel4.com/news/fgm-england-and-wales-home-office-survey-unicef-conference

16. https://www.theguardian.com/us-news/2016/dec/02/fgm-happened-to-me-in-white-midwest-america

17. https://theconversation.com/the-rise-and-fall-of-fgm-in-victorian-london-38327

18. https://www.the-tls.co.uk/sexual-mutilation-madness-and-the-media/

19. Rodriguez, S.B., 2014. *Female Circumcision and Clitoridectomy in the United States: A history of a medical treatment*. University of Rochester Press.

20. https://www.nytimes.com/1983/02/06/books/an-unlikely-analyst.html

21. https://www.menshealth.com.au/4-places-that-excite-her-more-than-the-g-spot

## Chapter Five: *The Orgasm, and Why Everything's Normal*

1. https://www.jahonline.org/article/S1054-139X(09)00485-6/fulltext

2. https://abcnews.go.com/Health/ReproductiveHealth/sex-study-female-orgasm-eludes-majority-women/story?id=8485289

3. Nagoski, E., 2015. *Come As You Are: The surprising new science that will transform your sex life*. Scribe UK.

4. https://www.ncbi.nlm.nih.gov/pubmed/11497209

5. https://www.theguardian.com/lifeandstyle/2016/nov/25/female-orgasm-research

6. https://www.theatlantic.com/health/archive/2011/05/why-cant-some-women-orgasm-neuroscience-might-finally-have-an-answer/238767/

7. https://www.theguardian.com/science/2005/jun/08/genetics.research

8. Herbenick D, Fu TC, Arter J, Sanders SA, Dodge B. Women's

experiences with genital touching, sexual pleasure, and orgasm: results from a US probability sample of women ages 18 to 94. *Journal of Sex & Marital Therapy.* 2017 Aug 8:1-2.

9. http://www.soc.ucsb.edu/sexinfo/article/clitoris
10. Friedan, B., 2010. *The Feminine Mystique.* Penguin Classics.
11. Freud, S., 1989. 'The psychology of women'. *New Introductory Lectures on Psycho-analysis.* WW Norton & Company.
12. https://www.cwluherstory.org/classic-feminist-writings-articles/myth-of-the-vaginal-orgasm
13. https://slutever.com/dr-barry-komisaruk/
14. https://link.springer.com/article/10.1007/s10508-017-0939-z
15. Fine, C., 2017. *Testosterone Rex: Unmaking the myths of our gendered minds.* Icon Books.
16. Gay, R., 2014. *Bad Feminist.* Corsair.
17. https://www.tandfonline.com/doi/full/10.1080/00224499.2017.1283484
18. https://www.psypost.org/2017/03/men-view-womens-orgasms-masculinity-achievement-study-finds-48360
19. https://www.omgyes.com/

## Chapter Six: *Appearances, and Looking in the Mirror*

1. https://www.self.com/story/yes-its-possible-to-tear-your-labia-and-its-more-common-than-youd-think
2. https://www.refinery29.com/pubic-hair-transplants
3. https://www.cosmopolitan.com/uk/body/news/a42147/half-young-women-uk-removing-all-pubic-hair/
4. https://www.nhs.uk/news/lifestyle-and-exercise/many-women-think-shaving-pubic-hair-is-hygienic
5. http://time.com/4590329/grooming-pubic-hair-sex-sti/
6. https://jezebel.com/instagram-deletes-designers-account-because-of-her-pub-1447051995
7. https://www.independent.co.uk/news/health/labiaplasty-vagina-surgery-cosmetic-procedure-plastic-study-international-society-aesthetic-plastic-a7837181.html
8. https://www.bbc.co.uk/news/health-40410459
9. Ibid.
10. https://www.theguardian.com/lifeandstyle/2011/oct/14/designer-vagina-surgery

11. Orenstein, P., 2016. *Girls & Sex: Navigating the complicated new landscape*. Oneworld Publications.

12. https://www.davidghozland.com/labiaplasty-comfort-aesthetics-spin-class/

## Chapter Seven: *Periods, and What Makes Them So Awful*

1. http://www.obgyn.net/young-women/first-menstruation-average-age-and-physical-signs

2. De Beauvoir, S., 1997. *The Second Sex*. Vintage Classics.

3. https://plan-uk.org/file/plan-uk-break-the-barriers-report-032018pdf/download?token=Fs-HYP3v

4. https://www.femmeinternational.org/our-work/the-issue/

5. https://www.popsci.com/science/article/2013-08/fyi-why-do-i-poop-more-when-i-have-my-period

6. https://www.theguardian.com/lifeandstyle/2016/mar/04/period-policy-asia-menstrual-leave-japan-women-work

7. Rooney, S., 2018. *Conversations with Friends*. Faber & Faber.

8. https://www.the-pool.com/arts-culture/books/2017/50/Sally-Rooney-on-periods-2017-conversations-with-friends

9. Steinem, G., 1985. *Outrageous Acts and Everyday Rebellions*. Flamingo.

10. https://www.nytimes.com/1982/03/07/magazine/dispelling-menstrual-myths.html

11. https://www.bustle.com/articles/80289-7-crazy-period-myths-from-history-because-people-once-thought-menstrual-blood-could-kill-crops

12. https://www.nytimes.com/2018/01/10/world/asia/nepal-woman-menstruation.html

13. https://plan-uk.org/file/plan-uk-break-the-barriers-report-032018pdf/download?token=Fs-HYP3v

14. http://www.bbc.com/news/uk-39266056

15. https://www.ncbi.nlm.nih.gov/pmc/articles/PMC4624246/

16. https://www.nytimes.com/2017/04/20/nyregion/pads-tampons-new-york-womens-prisons.html

17. https://plan-uk.org/file/plan-uk-break-the-barriers-report-032018pdf/download?token=Fs-HYP3v

18. https://www.theguardian.com/sport/shortcuts/2015/jan/21/menstruation-last-great-sporting-taboo

19. https://www.theguardian.com/society/2016/dec/12/
period-poverty-call-to-tackle-the-hidden-side-of-inequality

20. https://www.gov.uk/government/news/women-and-girls-set-to-
benefit-from-15-million-tampon-tax-fund

21. https://www.theguardian.com/business/2017/jul/28/tesco-
absorbs-tampon-tax-5-per-cent-vat-sanitary-products

22. https://twitter.com/LFC/status/1060985009471975426

23. http://www.vintageadbrowser.com/search?q=1935&page=6

24. https://www.prnewswire.com/news-releases/world-feminine-
hygiene-products-market-is-expected-to-reach-427-billion-by-
2022-575532151.html

25. https://www.london.gov.uk/sites/default/files/environment_
committee_-_plastic_unflushables.pdf

26. https://www.huffingtonpost.co.uk/entry/how-to-dispose-of-
tampons-and-pads-in-an-environmentally-friendly-way_uk_
5aec6e3be4b0c4f19321e67a

27. https://www.wen.org.uk/environmenstrualhistory/

## Chapter Eight: *Pain, As It Applies to Women*

1. Brockes, E., 2018. *An Excellent Choice: Panic and joy on my solo trip to motherhood*. Faber & Faber.

2. Jamison, L., 2014. Grand unified theory of female pain. *Virginia Quarterly Review*, 90(2), pp.114–28.

3. https://gupea.ub.gu.se/bitstream/2077/39196/1/gupea_2077_
39196_1.pdf; https://www.theatlantic.com/health/archive/
2015/10/emergency-room-wait-times-sexism/410515/

4. https://www.independent.co.uk/life-style/health-and-families/
health-news/how-sexist-stereotypes-mean-doctors-ignore-
womens-pain-a7157931.html

5. http://www.painmed.org/files/cecpw-policy-recommendations.pdf

6. https://www.ncbi.nlm.nih.gov/pmc/articles/PMC2745644//

7. http://www.bbc.com/future/story/20180518-the-inequality-in-how-
women-are-treated-for-pain

8. http://www.endwomenspain.org/

9. https://www.theguardian.com/society/2017/sep/06/listen-
to-women-uk-doctors-issued-with-first-guidance-on-
endometriosis

10. https://www.theguardian.com/society/2015/sep/28/endometriosis-
hidden-suffering-millions-women

11. https://edition.cnn.com/2016/03/22/health/endometriosis-fibroids-phthalates-dde-costs/index.html
12. https://www.vogue.com/article/lena-dunham-hysterectomy-vogue-march-2018-issue
13. https://www.instagram.com/p/BpCVOZElqPA/
14. https://www.theguardian.com/society/2004/jun/07/health.genderissues
15. https://news.virginia.edu/content/study-links-disparities-pain-management-racial-bias
16. https://www.jostrust.org.uk/node/451856
17. https://www.huffpost.com/entry/vulvodynia_b_1345062
18. https://www.cancerresearchuk.org/about-cancer/cervical-cancer/getting-diagnosed/screening/about
19. https://www.jostrust.org.uk/node/1075301
20. Ibid.
21. https://www.theguardian.com/society/2018/jul/20/cervical-cancer-testing-drive-will-aim-to-tackle-huge-surge-in-no-shows
22. https://www.bbc.co.uk/news/uk-england-45593583
23. https://assets.publishing.service.gov.uk/government/uploads/system/uploads/attachment_data/file/712239/HPV_primary_screening_leaflet.pdf
24. https://www.jostrust.org.uk/about-cervical-cancer/cervical-screening-smear-test-and-abnormal-cells/primary-hpv-testing/benefits
25. https://eveappeal.org.uk/gynaecological-cancers/?gclid=CjwKCA-jwpKveBRAwEiwAo4Pqm9JpkB_YLmMYywwR9pnD4xdIyjj-gLRIkt-GbYfCz4_utr0E-bR-tRoC5dgQAvD_BwE
26. https://www.cancerresearchuk.org/about-cancer/causes-of-cancer/infections-eg-hpv-and-cancer/hpv-and-cancer
27. https://academic.oup.com/bmb/article/114/1/5/246075

## Chapter Nine: *Fertility, Teaching It and Talking About It*

1. https://www.babycentre.co.uk/a1813/how-long-will-it-take-to-get-pregnant
2. https://www.nhs.uk/common-health-questions/pregnancy/how-long-does-it-usually-take-to-get-pregnant/
3. https://www.dailymail.co.uk/news/article-3677697/Warn-girls-nine-leaving-late-start-family-Expert-says-children-taught-fertility-young-age-ensure-remain-good-shape-baby.html#ixzz4DiFH0zYy

4. https://www.thetimes.co.uk/article/teach-girls-how-to-get-pregnant-say-doctors-8993hqbf9

5. https://www.nhs.uk/conditions/infertility/

6. https://theconversation.com/six-things-you-should-know-if-you-are-considering-freezing-your-eggs-94039

7. https://academic.oup.com/humupd/article/23/6/646/4035689

8. Martin, E., 1991. The egg and the sperm: How science has constructed a romance based on stereotypical male-female roles. *Signs: Journal of Women in Culture and Society*, 16(3), pp.485–501.

9. https://www.ncbi.nlm.nih.gov/pmc/articles/PMC196399/

10. https://www.theatlantic.com/magazine/archive/2013/07/how-long-can-you-wait-to-have-a-baby/309374/

Chapter Ten: *Getting Pregnant, and What Comes Next*

1. https://www.theguardian.com/society/2007/sep/12/health.medicineandhealth

2. https://www.nhs.uk/news/cancer/the-pill-provides-lifelong-protection-against-some-cancers/

3. https://www.independent.co.uk/voices/male-contraceptive-injection-successful-trial-halted-a7384601.html

4. https://www.thetimes.co.uk/article/pill-use-drops-as-women-put-faith-in-natural-cycles-app-6z27fw5q3

5. https://www.theguardian.com/technology/2018/jan/17/birth-control-app-natural-cycle-pregnancies

6. https://www.theguardian.com/society/2018/jul/21/colossally-naive-backlash-birth-control-app

7. https://www.bbc.co.uk/news/technology-45328965

8. https://www.thepharmaletter.com/article/oral-contraceptive-pills-market-to-reach-22-9-billion-by-2023-study

9. https://www.ons.gov.uk/peoplepopulationandcommunity/birthsdeathsandmarriages/conceptionandfertilityrates/bulletins/childbearingforwomenbornindifferentyearsenglandandwales/2016

10. https://www.huffingtonpost.co.uk/entry/quarter-of-all-pregnancies-end-in-abortion_uk_57343822e4b0f0f53e35bd7a

11. http://www.who.int/news-room/fact-sheets/detail/preventing-unsafe-abortion

12. https://assets.publishing.service.gov.uk/government/uploads/system/uploads/attachment_data/file/679028/Abortions_stats_England_Wales_2016.pdf

13. http://test.abortionrights.org.uk/did-you-know/
14. http://time.com/3956781/women-abortion-regret-reproductive-health/
15. https://www.nhs.uk/conditions/ectopic-pregnancy/
16. https://www.tommys.org/pregnancy-information/pregnancy-complications/baby-loss/miscarriage-information-and-support
17. http://edition.cnn.com/2011/HEALTH/06/09/miscarriage.not.fluke.ep/index.html
18. http://time.com/3849280/pregnancy-miscarriage/
19. https://www.imperial.ac.uk/news/175666/miscarriage-ectopic-pregnancy-trigger-post-traumatic-stress/
20. O'Farrell, M., 2018. *I Am, I Am, I Am.* Tinder Press.
21. Schiller, R., 2018. *Your No Guilt Pregnancy Plan.* Penguin Life.
22. https://theconversation.com/episiotomy-during-childbirth-not-just-a-little-snip-36062
23. Kitzinger, S. ed., 1981. *Episiotomy: Physical and emotional aspects.* National Childbirth Trust.
24. https://www.theguardian.com/lifeandstyle/2015/apr/12/sheila-kitzinger
25. Kitzinger, S. ed., 1981. *Episiotomy: Physical and emotional aspects.* National Childbirth Trust.
26. https://www.nhs.uk/conditions/caesarean-section/
27. http://www.birthrights.org.uk/wordpress/wp-content/uploads/2018/08/Final-Birthrights-MRCS-Report-2108.pdf
28. https://www.theguardian.com/society/2015/apr/10/caesarean-sections-medical-necessity-who
29. https://www.theguardian.com/society/2018/oct/11/use-of-caesarean-sections-growing-at-alarming-rate
30. https://www.theguardian.com/global-development/2018/sep/24/why-do-women-still-die-giving-birth
31. https://www.theguardian.com/lifeandstyle/2017/dec/07/better-medical-care-could-slash-uk-mortality-rate-during-pregnancy
32. https://www.bbc.co.uk/news/av/world-us-canada-42031800/why-do-so-many-us-women-die-giving-birth
33. https://vizhub.healthdata.org/fgh/
34. https://www.nytimes.com/2018/04/11/magazine/black-mothers-babies-death-maternal-mortality.html
35. https://www.nct.org.uk/life-parent/your-body-after-birth/incontinence-pregnancy-and-after-childbirth

36. https://www.mumsnet.com/campaigns/better-postnatal-care/birth-injuries-and-tears
37. https://www.hysterectomy-association.org.uk/information/why-do-i-need-a-hysterectomy/prolapse/
38. https://www.the-pool.com/health/wombs-etc/2018/14/Jennifer-Rigby-on-post-birth-vaginas

## Chapter Eleven: *The Vagina and Menopause*

1. https://pudding.cool/2017/03/film-dialogue/index.html
2. https://www.bbc.co.uk/news/entertainment-arts-22554217
3. https://www.telegraph.co.uk/news/bbc/11349310/BBC-had-an-informal-policy-to-discriminate-against-older-women-say-peers.html
4. https://www.nhs.uk/conditions/menopause/
5. https://www.health.harvard.edu/blog/menopause-related-hot-flashes-night-sweats-can-last-years-201502237745
6. Henpicked, 2018. *Menopause: The change for the better*. Green Tree.
7. Greer, G., 2018. *The Change*. Bloomsbury Publishing.
8. https://www.nhs.uk/conditions/menopause/symptoms/
9. https://www.ncbi.nlm.nih.gov/pmc/articles/PMC3735281/
10. Greer, G., 2018. *The Change*. Bloomsbury Publishing.
11. https://www.ncbi.nlm.nih.gov/pmc/articles/PMC3735281/
12. Ibid.
13. https://www.telegraph.co.uk/news/2016/05/19/half-of-women--too-embarrassed-to-speak-to-doctor-about-menopaus/
14. https://www.theguardian.com/books/2014/apr/11/jeanette-winterson-can-you-stop-the-menopause
15. Greer, G., 2018. *The Change*. Bloomsbury Publishing.
16. https://jamanetwork.com/journals/jama/fullarticle/195120
17. https://www.womens-health-concern.org/help-and-advice/factsheets/hrt-the-history/
18. Ibid.
19. https://www.nice.org.uk/news/article/women-with-symptoms-of-menopause-should-not-suffer-in-silence
20. https://www.telegraph.co.uk/news/health/news/11989679/New-NHS-advice-means-number-of-women-on-HRT-could-double.html
21. https://jamanetwork.com/journals/jama/fullarticle/2653735

22. https://www.theguardian.com/society/2017/sep/15/hrt-hormone-replacement-therapy-wont-kill-you-but-menopausal-women-still-face-a-difficult-decision

23. https://www.theguardian.com/books/2014/apr/11/jeanette-winterson-can-you-stop-the-menopause

24. https://www.nhs.uk/conditions/hormone-replacement-therapy-hrt/

25. https://www.fda.gov/newsevents/newsroom/pressannouncements/ucm615130.htm

26. https://www.callyourgirlfriend.com/episodes#/believe-womens-pain/

27. https://www.itv.com/news/2016-11-23/quarter-of-women-going-through-menopause-considered-leaving-work/

## Chapter Twelve: *Does My Vagina Define Me?*

1. https://www.elle.com/culture/career-politics/a14059/transgender-women-body-image/

2. https://www.stonewall.org.uk/help-advice/glossary-terms#t

3. Lester, CN, 2017. *Trans Like Me*. Virago Publishing.

4. https://www.channel4.com/news/factcheck/factcheck-qa-how-many-children-are-going-to-gender-identity-clinics-in-the-uk

5. https://assets.publishing.service.gov.uk/government/uploads/system/uploads/attachment_data/file/721642/GEO-LGBT-factsheet.pdf

6. http://endtransdiscrimination.org/report.html

7. https://www.gires.org.uk/wp-content/uploads/2014/08/AIAUSatisfactionAuditJune2008.pdf

8. https://broadly.vice.com/en_us/article/evq43w/buck-angel-how-learning-to-love-my-vagina-affirmed-my-manhood

9. https://broadly.vice.com/en_us/article/59jgkb/transgender-vaginoplasty-juno-roche-essay

10. https://www.thejournal.ie/poll-what-influenced-your-vote-4036674-May2018/

11. https://www.stonewall.org.uk/lgbt-britain-trans-report

12. https://www.theproudtrust.org/resources/research-and-guidance-by-other-organisations/lgbt-youth-homelessness-a-uk-national-scoping-of-cause-prevalence-response-and-outcome/

13. https://www.gires.org.uk/wp-content/uploads/2016/02/BAME_Inclusivity.pdf

14. https://twitter.com/JanelleMonae/status/983894793712553984

### REFERENCES

15. https://twitter.com/TessaThompson_x/status/983795559743049728
16. https://broadly.vice.com/en_us/article/mbxxqp/janelle-monae-pynk-video-saved-pussy-power-from-white-feminism
17. https://www.vice.com/en_nz/article/j5gk8p/is-the-vagina-monologues-still-woke
18. http://www.who.int/genomics/gender/en/index1.html
19. Adichie, C.N., 2013. We should all be feminists. TedxEuston.